GERONTOLOGIC HUMAN RESOURCES

GERONTOLOGIC HUMAN RESOURCES

The Role of the Paraprofessional

Joan M. Settin, Ph.D.

Program on Aging,
Bangor Mental Health Institute
Bangor, Maine.

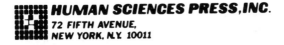

HUMAN SCIENCES PRESS, INC.
72 FIFTH AVENUE,
NEW YORK, N.Y. 10011

Library of Congress Cataloging in Publication Data

Settin, Joan M.
  Gerontologic human resources.

  Bibliography: p. 145
  Includes index.
  1. Aged—Care and Hygiene. 2. Aged—Mental health. 3. Allied health personnel. I. Title. [DNLM. 1. Aging. 2. Geriatrics—Manpower. 3. Allied health personnel. WT 21 S495g]
  RA564.8.S47   618.97′0233   LC 81-6315
  ISBN 0-89885-042-8   AACR2

CONTENTS

PREFACE

The central theme of this book is that health care for the aging should be no less progressive than health care for any other segment of society. Social policies reflecting a view of the aging as an "out group" have in the past made it less likely for adequate attention to be focused on training staff to work with the aging. As a result, the aging have received primarily custodial care frequently based upon myths and stereotypes concerning the aging process. However true, this type of fault within the system analysis does not offer a practical short-term solution to the current service crisis among health personnel working with the aging. It is felt that utilization of an available human resource, that of the paraprofessional, does offer such a practical solution.

Paraprofessionals have been referred to as auxiliary personnel, aides, indigenous workers, nonprofessionals. They are welcomed by some professionals as additional intervention agents, and have been accorded real responsibilities in line with their training; others have not been regarded as having the requisite skills and have been assigned tasks of material preparation, cleanup, and custodial chores. Health planners have grappled with the problem of role definition, training direction, and career development for paraprofessionals, while individual professionals continue to view them as a mixed blessing.

There is a danger in advocating the utilization of paraprofessionals with the aging, and it resides in ageist attitudes held by health professionals about treatment for the aging. This danger is to make the erroneous assumption that because paraprofessionals are less well educated and thus less prestigeous than professionals, the populations with whom they work must be deserving of less professional intervention. The point is that paraprofessionals and professionals provide different services, they do not replace one another's services, and both types of services are needed by aging clients.

The trainers of future health paraprofessionals will be allied health professionals. This book is intended for those who desire an overview of gerontological health-care issues as they relate to paraprofessionals, in order to foster an awareness of the realities and to dispel some of the myths surrounding aging in America. For paraprofessionals to be able to intervene effectively, it is important that the kind of training they receive be carefully articulated. If so, they will (a) knowledgeably upgrade interpersonal and helping skills necessary to appropriate therapeutic intervention with the aging and (b) understand the parameters of their involvement.

This book took shape in several stages. What began as a proposal for a training school for gerontologic paraprofessionals evolved into a curriculum for "geriatric technicians", became an in-service training manual for mental health therapy aides on a geriatric service in a state psychiatric institute, and finally reached its present form. The primary motivation throughout this process was the prototypical aging individual who fails to receive needed treatment because of lack of options, ageism, or frank neglect. Additional motivation was furnished by a belief that formation of positive expectations leads to positive experiences with the aging, and by a conviction that the future of allied health services for the aging lies in a prevention model of community health wherein trained paraprofessionals play a central role as intervention agents, participant observers, environmental designers, advocates, and case managers. Lastly, I have been motivated by the aging people in my family who were responsible for my early views of nursing homes, hospitals, and other institutions. Their late life struggles with the American health-care system helped to crystalize my views concerning the drastic need for alternatives for the aging, both within and without institutions.

J.M.S.

Chapter 1

DEVELOPMENT OF THE PARAPROFESSIONAL RESOURCE

An Historical Overview

By original definition, the paraprofessional is regarded as one who relieves professionals with any number of preparatory, organizational, and supervisory duties, freeing them to carry out professional duties. Such a definition is based upon a concept of service provision restricted to formal intervention modalities. A less traditional point of view defines the paraprofessional as any individual who serves the purpose of providing health services without having been professionally trained (Sobey, 1970). More radical advocates for paraprofessional health workers have even taken the extremist view that the paraprofessional will eventually become the primary disseminator of services within the allied health field (Durlak, 1973; Danish and Augelli, 1976; Jeger, 1976).

The American approach to health care has largely ignored the notion of preventive health care practiced by many other countries such as England, for example, in which comprehensive support networks rely heavily upon paraprofessionals for service delivery.

A future outlook must expand to include alternatives to traditional service-delivery personnel in allied health fields. For example, critics of our traditional health-care systems have long argued for the expansion of community support services. As this occurs, there will exist a service crisis within these alternatives to institutionalization.

While considerable attention is being devoted to policy planning for the aging, there continues to be little attention drawn to projected human-resource needs, which will necessarily arise from reorganization of health-service networks in the future. Part of the explanation for this lack of attention lies in the unwillingness of the professional community to delegate responsibility to non-title-holding health workers. Another part of this unwillingness involves the fact that paraprofessionals working in the field of aging have traditionally been geriatric aides. Usually working in an institutional environment where the aging patient assumes perhaps the lowest priority on the patient hierarchy, the geriatric aide has acquired the role of primary custodial care provider. And, because the aging patient has been so consistently ignored, implementation of training programs in gerontology has lagged far behind programs in other disciplines.

This unwillingness is gradually diminishing with the realization that professionals are overloaded in the performance of their technical duties by nontechnical activities that conceivably could be performed by other trained staff. In addition, the changing face of the American health-care system, coupled with the recent interest stimulated in socioenvironmental problems of the aging, has shifted emphasis toward alternatives to institutionalization. The paraprofessional trainee in geriatrics (*geriatrics* defined as the study and treatment of the diseases of old age), receives training primarily in abnormal processes, which will not be sufficient for future job directions for paraprofessionals working with the aging in which normal as well as abnormal processes will be implicated. Further, it is becoming more widely accepted that "the greatest benefit would accrue to society if non-professionals . . . could be drawn from a segment of society that normally would not be contributing to the economy and might even be a drain on society's resources" (Zax and Specter, 1974). Such individuals could include the retired, persons looking for new career directions, or the unemployed. That post-secondary education does not always offer practical training opportunities, particularly where the cost of four or more years of college may be prohibitive, is an issue of growing concern. These are but a few of the compelling reasons in support of the use of paraprofessionals in gerontology. As a result, the paraprofessional's role in working with the aging is rapidly expanding from one concerned exclusively with the medical or custodial orientation of geriatrics into one concerned with the study of the general phenomena of aging that is gerontology.

A primary goal of preventive aging health care is intervention in normal aging processes with the goal of forestalling unnecessary decline. Because preventive community health services are widely accepted as desirable intervention strategies, particularly for the aging segment of society, it is hoped that paraprofessionals will someday be working in the community to help prevent disability from occurring. Where minor disability exists, Kahn's (1975) principle of least intervention implies that community support networks, if available, will provide the appropriate work setting for paraprofessionals. Where major disability exists, paraprofessionals will provide a needed human resource within institutional or alternate care settings.

In the early 1960s with the advent of community health legislation and increased allocation of resources, a service crisis did indeed exist in the American health-care system. Inadequate numbers of health professionals created a burgeoning need for supportive staff. Consequently, a shift toward increased utilization of paraprofessionals took place, a change manifested, for example, by relabeling hospital attendants "psychiatric" or "therapy" aides. Unfortunately, relabeling did not entail retraining, with the result that these paraprofessionals rapidly diminished in both effectiveness and popularity and their utilization by the 1970s was seriously curtailed. Even for adequately trained paraprofessionals, lack of job advancement, prestige, and reinforcement on the job stifled their enthusiasm and allowed their skills to fall into disuse.

This situation corresponded with an overabundance of degree-holding professionals in the job market who responded defensively to the notion that paraprofessionals might appear in large numbers. The oft-quoted rationale for utilization of paraprofessionals, that of shortages in service providers, is thus not entirely accurate. It would be more accurate to say that experimentation in the delivery of health services has created new jobs requiring a reappraisal of the paraprofessional potential.

PARAPROFESSIONALS AS PSYCHOSOCIAL INTERVENTION AGENTS

While paraprofessionals in primarily custodial and physical rehabilitative areas (e.g., nursing aides, physical-therapy aides, etc.) have been fairly well integrated into the health team, the mental-health paraprofessional continues to occupy a more controversial role. There has thus been a call for assessment of the effectiveness of paraprofessionals in the psychosocial area. Within psychiatric institutions, the paraprofessional psychiatric aid is one of the most important members of the therapeutic team. Beginning in the early 1960s, Appleby (1963) demonstrated that psychiatric aides functioning as "models" produced a significant improvement compared with controls in the level of daily functioning of chronic inpatients. Carkhuff and Traux (1965), Ellsworth (1968), and Saunders, Smith, and Weinman (1969) found that lay personnel provided more effective intervention than a comparison control, or than comparison staff (Rappaport, Chinsky and Cohen, 1971; Poser, 1966).

In the outpatient and community sector, community adults (Mendel and Rapport, 1963) and psychiatric aides (Bergin and Solomon, 1963) were found to be appropriate, well accepted, and effective as intervention agents with normal aging adults. Marx, Test, and Stein (1973) found that former hospital workers in autonomous community settings were more beneficial than controls in effecting change in chronic patients. Cowen, Liebowitz, and Liebowitz (1968) and Hallowitz and Riessman (1967) successfully trained indigenous community residents to function as community mental-health aides.

The dependent variable "effectiveness" used so often in studies on paraprofessional performance can mean many things. It may refer to acceptance of the role of the paraprofessional by staff (perceived role congruency), or it may relate to organizational dimensions such as reliability, accountability, trustworthiness, and so on. The issue is not whether paraprofessionals are more or less effective than other individuals (e.g., professionals), but whether they are differently effective because their roles, attitudes, and abilities are different. In other words, it is quite another story to measure effectiveness in terms of outcome for the client, or observed constructive personal change. In evaluating comparative studies of paraprofessionals versus professionals, it is thus important to look at the yardstick by which outcome is measured. For example, if the dependent outcome variable is "motivation to attend group therapy," it may be that liking for the group leader is the significant variable, not necessarily a change in client level of motivation.

The theme running throughout is that some intervention is better than no intervention, and in some cases paraprofessionals can be more effective than professionals. However pedestrian these results may seem, they do provide empirical justification for using paraprofessionals both within and without institutions for intervention with so-called chronic psychiatric patients. Importantly, when these studies are analyzed into groups of trained versus untrained paraprofessionals, it becomes apparent that the trained paraprofessionals are responsible for the significant positive results in a large percentage of the cases. "The multiplicity of data garnered by different investigators, with different biases and employing different research tools, add up to quite a convincing picture. This is not to say that paraprofessionals always or necessarily better the performance of the agencies, but frequently they do, and with appropriate training they can improve the service considerably" (Riessman, 1971).

PARAPROFESSIONAL TRAINING IN ALLIED HEALTH

Paraprofessionals have traditionally received little or no training prior to entering their work setting. However, with recent research stressing the importance of training, the role of the trained paraprofessional has achieved legitimacy and has been largely influenced by industrial and organizational psychologists who have for years insisted that behavior is composed of identifiable "trainable" components. For example, it is now recognized that job effectiveness relates to such variables as need achievement, communication skills, and attitudinal congruence with expectations. Training programs taking these variables into account have proliferated in recent years, and particular emphasis is now being placed upon the need for systematic training for the health paraprofessional in "other-enhancement" areas characteristic of effective interpersonal interactions.

Debate has taken place over the relative merits of didactic versus experiential training techniques for the paraprofessional. Principles common to most effective training programs (in the form of trainer instructions) are: (1) teaching observable behaviors; (2) modeling both desired and undesired behaviors, then practicing reverse role play; (3) providing immediate, corrective feedback in a nonevaluative climate; and (4) discussing feelings and attitudes toward the target population and the role of the paraprofessional. It is generally accepted that a multi-modal training approach combining modeling techniques, role play, and discussion with didactic presentation is an effective training strategy.

Stone and Vance (1976) evaluated alternate paraprofessional training techniques of instruction, modeling, rehearsal, and the combined conditions (instruction and modeling, instruction and rehearsal, modeling and rehearsal, instruction, modeling, and rehersal) against a no-training control. Immediately following training, participants (48 undergraduate psychology students) responded to 16 stimulus statements judged on an empathy scale. Two weeks following training, participants were placed in a role-play situation, an interview requiring empathic communication skills, and were evaluted. Results indicated that any of the combined (e.g., multi-modal) techniques produced higher levels of empathy in paraprofessionals than did any single technique, with modeling producing a critical effect. Thus, one primary component of training helping skills, empathy, can be conceptualized as requiring both understanding of the content of the helping skill and practice in using the skill.

Danish and Hauer's (1973) helping-skills training program outlines "core" conditions that are prerequisite to helpful intervention, including positive regard and genuineness in addition to empathic understanding. Six stages integrate three components necessary for acquisition of effective helping behaviors: understanding of one's self, knowledge of helping skills, and experience in applying these skills. Paraprofessionals are led through six progressive stages: (1) understanding one's needs to be a paraprofessional; (2) using effective nonverbal behavior; (3) using effective verbal behavior; (4) using effective self-involving behavior; (5) understanding others' communications; and (6) establishing effective helping relationships. Although there have been several such excellent programs for generalized skill training, there have been few that specifically address the aging client. One paraprofessional training program (Settin, 1979b), implemented with therapy aides on a geriatric admissions unit of a psychiatric center, used primarily experiential group techniques. Emphasis was placed on communication and sensitivity training, using situation specific topics in gerontology as illustrative material (see Appendix I).

It has been suggested that paraprofessionals are effective health-service providers because of their similarity to the client, where the helping team includes: "workers from the same milieu as the clients served by the team, and these workers could well be much more successful than the fully qualified professional in making contact with potential clients, in motivating them, and in interpreting the agency to the client. Where they have been well trained and well supervised, indigenous leaders have made important contributions which cannot be made by anyone else. There are dimensions of expression, voice inflection, gesture, body language, which are almost instantly recognizable as signs of class and ethnic origin. The indigenous leader can communicate instantly to this suspicious and distrustful client, avoiding noblesse oblige, in a way that many middle class professionals cannot do" (Gordon, 1965).

However, widespread success of Danish and Hauer's (1973) training program would suggest that paraprofessionals need not necessarily be similar to the population served; rather, they need to possess basic helping skills that may augment personal characteristics of the paraprofessional, such as warmth or interest in providing intervention (Settin, 1979a). Recognition that personal characteristics have great impact on the allied health paraprofessional's effectiveness has resulted in the development of the GAIT (Group Assessment of Interpersonal Traits) screening device (Goodman, 1972). This strategy of comparatively evaluating potential paraprofessionals focuses upon clarity of communication as a primary determinant of effective helping behavior. This screening device may be used both as a training tool and as a feedback-giving mechanism.

The nature of the training appropriate for paraprofessionals depends not only on technique and personal characteristics but also varies according to the nature of the population to receive services. It is fortunate that the very target population, the neglected aging within and without institutions, are also those who can most benefit from paraprofessional services (Hickey, 1976). This neglect has in part been a reflection of the widespread myth that aging clients are less responsive to therapeutic intervention than younger clients. The result is that paraprofessionals are often not prepared for other than custodial work, and are too frequently trained by professionals who themselves may find it distasteful to work with the aging.

There has been much complaining done by professionals about the alleged lack of enthusiasm on the part of paraprofessional staff (e.g., therapy aides) despite their training, and the need for staff motivation and morale boosting. This frankly bespeaks lack of sensitivity or lack of insight, or both, on the part of professionals. It is a fact that trained paraprofessionals enter their field with great enthusiasm for their job, enthusiasm that is quickly squelched by lack of reinforcement. For example, mental-health therapy aides are trained to provide therapeutic intervention, yet upon entering the job setting they discover that their duties are largely custodial and that a floor's shine is more important than a client's affect. They are reinforced for this custodial work and are not reinforced for socializing on the ward with clients. Furthermore, they are not only ignored by elitist professionals, but are excluded from input into treatment planning for clients (an area where they clearly could contribute important client information due to opportunity for observation and interaction). A specific paraprofessional training segment should thus be preparation for such antiparaprofessional sentiment and for the reality of "working within the system." Additional areas for exploration related to this topic are prevention of staff burnout due to early disillusionment, and maintenance of internal motivation through alternate sources of reinforcement.

Reinforcement in the form of feedback has been studied by Panyon, Boozer, and Morris (1970), who trained 34 hospital therapy aides in behavior-change techniques. Staff were asked to keep daily baseline performance records for assigned clients needing training in improving self-management in areas of dressing, toileting, and self-feeding generally referred to as Activities of Daily Living (ADL) Skills. Evaluation of therapy-aide performance by the resident psychologist consisted of tabulating the percent of skill-training sessions implemented with clients. Feedback was given in written form, including rank-ordering, which compared one ward's performance with other participating wards, to all staff following completion of baseline. Immediately following training, the percent of sessions with clients was high, but steadily decreased week by week with no feedback. Providing reinforcement to staff, in the form of feedback, resulted in a significant increase in the percent of self-help sessions provided to clients.

Paraprofessionals can be effectively trained to use "curative" techniques such as interviewing to promote communication through reflection, role playing to promote production of appropriate behavior through imitation, and psychodrama to promote insight through catharsis. These techniques are applicable to all target populations. It may be that training needs additionally to be practically geared toward specific target populations, based upon the notion that different populations (e.g., the aging) may respond much more strongly to therapist attitudes toward aging rather than to different techniques of intervention.

For these reasons, it is important to match the personal career goals of paraprofessionals with (a) general training in helping skills and (b) specific training in gerontology. Health professionals and paraprofessionals alike cannot be expected to be totally unbiased or to have facility with all clients. Ageism, defined by Butler (1969) as a "deep seated uneasiness on the part of the young and middle aged . . . a personal repulsion to and distaste for growing old, disease, disability, and fear of powerlessness, uselessness, and death" has many roots, yet the possibility cannot be excluded that dislike for working with the aging stems from a perfectly legitimate preference for other-than-aging target populations.

The need for new paraprofessionals is undeniable at this point in time. A gerontologic paraprofessional in the hospital system could perform many of the functions normally done, for example, by a practical nurse pertaining to special problems of the aging client. In the community setting, one issue of primary concern for the aging at high risk for physical and emotional illness is that of utilization of existing clinic services. The effectiveness of the "neighborhood representative" or the "family health worker" suggests that paraprofessionals could effect great improvement in this area (Haskell, 1979). An innovative new role for the paraprofessional might be that of geriatric family health paraprofessional, a blend of social advocate and service expediter (interpreting services offered to aging residents, dealing with complaints, making referrals to appropriate authorities), acting as a caseworker (dealing with individual problems and providing follow-up), crisis interventionalist, and educator.

Chapter 2

SOCIAL REALITIES OF AGING

AGE CATEGORIZATION

U.S. Bureau of the Census figures for 1980 place the population of the age of 65 at a little over 24 million persons of whom roughly 9 million will be age 75 and over (Siegel, 1972). The 65-74 age group, which in 1980 represents roughly 9.3% of the total U.S. population, is estimated by the year 2000 to have increased by fully 23%; the 75+ age group is projected to increase by 60%. This large increase is partially due to advances in medical science; many of the disease processes that contribute to the present mortality rate, particularly infant mortality, are being decreased in severity and frequency of occurrence. In addition to advances in medical science, social factors such as the increased acceptability of family planning, indicate that the aging population is actually growing faster than the younger population at this time.

Compared with the younger population, the aging population consists of greater numbers of women than men due to the greater longevity of females. This population also has a comparably lower household income, the median being $4,800 compared with

$12,400 for the 18–64 age group (McCluskey, 1978). Contrary to popular belief, aging persons are found to be living in nursing and adult homes only 4% of the time, and in mental institutions only 1% of the time (Libow, 1973). This means that fully 95% of the aging in America live in the community, and implies that the percentage of aging persons who are functionally totally incapacitated is insignificant compared with those who continue to function in total or near total health.

Health statistics concerning the community aging vary from study to study. One of the reasons for the wide variance in these statistics concerning the segment of our society collectively referred to as "the aging" is the great heterogeneity of this population. The age of 65 represents one of many age markers in a lifetime that can withstand two or more additional decades of growth, and there are distinct differences in social, physical, and emotional aging between a 65- and a 78-year-old person. For this reason, health professionals have begun to base epidemiological statistics upon "young-old" (65–74) and "old-old" (75+) age categories (Neugarten and Havighurst, 1976).

It may be that a focus on the special problems of the aging (which was largely responsible for the emergence of the field of gerontology devoted entirely to the aging) is no longer a productive or necessarily even an appropriate concept. In other words, age segregation, once a necessary step toward drawing attention to the needs of this neglected population, may actually have the effect of emphasizing pathology rather than normalcy while de-emphasizing individual differences. Particularly in the health professions, aging is now being viewed in terms of life span development (rather than in segments such as "young-old") in which individual differences primarily determine the outcome of the person's health status.

CYCLE OF DECLINE

Despite individual differences, the population aged 65 and over continue to have in common the experience of a socioeconomic environment that is critically different from that experienced by "younger" members of society. For example, major socioeconomic links in the pattern leading to continued well-being for the aging are: (a) ownership or control of private property and centralization of resources, (b) command of strategic knowledge of the culture, (c) maintenance of kinship structures, (d) institutionalization of obligations to societal members (Rosow, 1962). As is painfully obvious, these links in the chain are so weakened for the majority of today's aging that not even social legislation can reverse the cycle of decline precipitated by loss of income through retirement. Although most aging persons own their homes, their income is no longer adequate in meeting the rising costs of maintenance. While the aging do command a knowledge of the culture, increasing technology is making their strategic knowledge obsolete. Kinship structures are changing rapidly and many aging persons have not established folk-support networks consisting of informal social relations with friends, neighbors, or social-group members to replace the traditional family support structures. In short, the majority of aging are segregated from their accustomed social roles, a situation that results in rolelessness and feeds into a cycle of decline.

Characterized by disuse leading to inactivity, low morale, and subsequent illness, the cycle of decline is difficult to reverse once begun. A typical cycle might follow a pattern of: (a) exclusion from accustomed social roles, (b) decrease in self-esteem, (c) failing physical and emotional health, (d) dependence upon institutions for care, (e) further decrease in self-esteem and social stigmatization, (f) disorientation, (g) resignation, (h) labeling by others as "untreatable," and (i) vegetation and/or death (Barnes, Sack, and Shore, 1973). Aging persons caught up in this cycle are likely to be held responsible at stages (e), (f), and (g) for their decline. Such a "victim blaming" (Ryan, 1971) approach, for example, would be the institutionalized aging person who is incontinent for reason of organic brain syndrome but scolded by staff for urinating in bed.

The notion that decline and deterioration are synonymous

with age deserves some comment. A labeling bias perspective assumes that the aging are no more intrinsically weakened or deteriorated than members of other age groups, but are labeled as more deteriorated based upon some negative perception of aging. Since there is no evidence that the aging become physically or psychologically incapacitated to any significant extent unless they are subject to an abnormal disease process, it can be argued that the healthy aging person is no more predisposed toward acquisition of negative health attributes (such as suspiciousness, for example) than the younger person. In other words, given equal opportunity and equal capability, the fact of chronological age alone is an insufficient condition for differential treatment. Yet, aging individuals continue to be blamed for their supposed decline and deterioration.

It might be more appropriate to view this cycle as affected not so much by personal characteristics of the aging person as by adverse environments. For example, poverty, pollution, lack of exercise, poor nutrition, or inadequate folk-support networks limit an individual's ability to cope with stress. The cumulative effect of a lifetime of stress is undoubtedly more important than the stress generated by age-linked social traumas (Lowenthal, 1968). Thus, the lifelong pattern of dealing with stress includes coping mechanisms and social support networks interacting to form an adaptive mode. The absence of this adaptive pattern, in combination with accumulated stress and inadequate social support, could cause the aging person to "break down" and have to leave the community setting temporarily (but usually permanently) for a total-support environment. There is increasing evidence that aging persons institutionalized more than once usually stay there. Typically, for every one problem with which the person enters the institution, there emerge two problems shortly after entry. This multiple pathology may result from infection, drug effects, trauma, lack of activity, and depression, to name but a few factors which may lead to the need for continuing institutionalization. Traditional total-support environments are the nursing home and/or health-related facility, or the psychiatric center.

The nursing home is the most frequently utilized alternate environment, since on the surface it appears to offer multi-level care under one roof. In reality, not all nursing homes include health-related facilities and not all operate with the goal of returning the individual to the community. The psychiatric center's focus too often excludes from importance the physical components of illness, which may lead to neglect of potentially reversible problems. Such total institutions, clearly inappropriate under most circumstances, house a vast number of aging persons who should be receiving treatment elsewhere but have neither the means, opportunity, nor support to do so. Such persons have typically entered the institution years ago when no alternate treatment modalities were available. Alcoholics, vagrants, drug users, criminals, the blind, the paraplegic, the diabetic, and many others found themselves inappropriately placed in psychiatric facilities.

The process of institutionalization may begin with a series of interrelated social problems combined with a mild physical problem, as is described by the following case history:

> Mr. T., who retired at age 65, is now aged 67, and widowed. He and his wife had no children. He lives alone in a two-story house, where the nearest shopping center cannot be reached by foot and there is no public transportation. Because he has no income other than his social security and rent from tenants, he has financial difficulties that increase with inflation. He had relied greatly upon his wife for companionship and housekeeping. He now hardly ever goes out, but sits in front of the TV most of the day, becoming increasingly depressed. While on the way to the mailbox one winter, he falls and breaks his hip.

This person was hospitalized for the hip fracture and transfered to a nursing home for three months of "rehabilitation." While in the nursing home, his personal affairs were left unattended and his tenants moved. He became increasingly depressed about his life prospects and depended upon the nursing-home staff for activities he had easily performed for himself while living in the community. He has a certain future of continued institutionalization ahead.

The aging person who can afford to continue to live in the community should do well compared with the institutionalized person whose declining health status impedes continued community living. Yet there is much undiagnosed emotional disorder among the community aging (Morrice, 1977), to the point where the aging white male with a drinking problem is considered one of the most likely candidates for suicide (Eisdorfer, 1972), accounting for 28% of the total suicides in the United States in 1966, the rate rising steadily with increasing age (U.S. Vital Statistics, 1968). At highest risk for suicide is the retired or unemployed isolated city-dwelling male (Gardner, Bahn, and Mack, 1963). Rolelessness, a result of exclusion from accustomed social roles, carries with it the seeds of emotional disorder. When no demand exists for what have previously been central roles, that member of society becomes obsolete.

Forced Obsolescence

Unlike some cultures in which the aging are integral components of the family structure for purposes of acculturation (training younger members in familial and societal history, mores, rituals, and providing cultural continuity), American society allows younger family or nonfamily members to fill this role. Duties of parenthood end earlier in a nuclear family than would be the case in an extended family, such that grandparents and even parents occupy an increasingly marginal position in their children's lives. Objective factors brought about by urbanization, such as smaller living space, make it more difficult to accomodate aging relatives. It is thus the case that social relationships, which had previously constituted an important source of social control in the extended family structure and which had constrained the upwardly mobile younger members, are becoming increasingly superficial.

Particularly for the aging male, loss of status due to retirement from the occupational role is primarily responsible for fostering current stereotypes of the aging (including aging persons' own self-beliefs) of nonproductivity. An additional social factor bearing upon the aging person's loss of status is the emergence of a youth-culture ideology predicated upon the notion of novel consumption. Industrial societies reinforce this conception of nonproductivity by viewing the worth of their members in terms of work productivity. In the 1930's, the economics of cost effectiveness was illustrated by Franklin D. Roosevelt's intention to revitalize the Supreme Court with younger men who did not suffer from "a lowered mental and physical vigor which leads men to avoid examination of complicated and changed situations . . ." (Gruman, 1978). As industrialization and automation increased, the value of the older worker decreased; the creation of the Social Security Act virtually insured obsolescence at the age of 65.

Other examples of systems that increase expendability are some modern-day workmen's compensation (Braginsky, 1978) and Medicare/Medicaid policies, which encourage a sick role by making more income available for the infirm aging. Even when the individual over 65 is fortunate enough to find employment, there still exists a ceiling for earnings, past which one-half of every social security dollar is withdrawn for every income dollar declared. In other words, persons over the age of 65 who earn more than their quotas must forfeit $1.00 in benefits for every $2.00 earned that year in excess of the current $5500.00 quota.

A realistic look at retirement discloses the fact that it fulfills expectations in less than half the cases (Harris, 1975), and for many means depression, impoverishment, and disenfranchisement (Corman, 1973). Aging persons often retire to communities located far from their neighborhood where full services (including medical and recreational facilites) are promised but not forthcoming. Critics of retirement communities point out that this type of "total environment" serves to further segregate the aging, rather than to promote integration of this age group into society. In fact, there are numerous cases where aging persons retire to such communities for a year and decide to move back to their old neighborhoods after finding the retirement community alienating, antiseptic, or just plain boring. In other words, it may be more desirable for the maintenance of health and life satisfaction for people to struggle but retain the flavor of life, than to be transplanted into an unfamiliar and too homogeneous environment. With widespread loss of social roles, most aging need to retain neighborhood ties, however marginal, and to marshall their resources against poverty. The fact is that full retirement, once heralded as a panacea, is now an unaffordable luxury for most aging.

The situation is bleak for those who prefer not to retire but cannot compete with more highly trained young workers. On-the-job experience has become less valuable with the advent of automation. Inducements to retire from within the occupational system, such as pension plan "benefits," conceal the fact that the job market solicits early retirement of the aging worker. It is thus in the best interests of business to perpetuate those myths accentuating the nonproductive aspects of aging, such as decrement in reaction time, deterioration of the visual and auditory sense, or memory loss. While losses in physiological functioning are surely evidenced to some extent with aging process, the aging are well able to compensate for most normal age-related losses: "The nature and extent of these changes are such, however, that at least 86% of persons over 65 remain sufficiently mobile and in the community managing to cope with the demands of everyday life" (Weg, 1973). This physiological decline argument is thus no longer a viable excuse for ending occupational productivity through forced retirement practices.

As can be seen, social policies affecting the aging may actually make it more profitable to be retired or unemployed or, until recently, unmarried (an example of the latter was the decrease in Social Security payments to married aging persons). This is ironic in light of the fact that loss of occupational status and loss of meaningful personal relationships have been identified as the two most serious social problems confronting the aging in America today. "The fact that people grow old does not in itself account for many of the changes in mood and behavior observed in old age. The role changes that signify permanent detachment from society's two principle institutional systems—the nuclear family and the occupational system—are far more important factors than physical changes" (Blau, 1973). These role changes seriously affect the attitudes held toward the aging, including prejudicial ageist attitudes on the part of health professionals and paraprofessionals. Individual prejudices are amenable to change on some level through the personal efforts of the individual holding those biases. However, in the case of institutional discrimination, change involves reorganization on a structural level. It is likely that individual prejudices would not persist were they not sanctioned by institutional norms. Understanding the process whereby such attitudes are formed should facilitate some attitude change.

A social-role analysis of aging in America suggests that institutional discrimination may in fact precede individual prejudice. For example, the stereotyping process affecting the aging occurs as meaningful roles are denied to this group (e.g., through blanket retirement practices). These aging members of society are then expendable and are singled out for devaluation. As they become less a part of mainstream society, they are gradually assigned to increasingly peripheral roles (McTavish, 1971; Brubaker and Powers, 1976; Solomon, 1978). The labeling process, applying pejorative terminology to this devalued segment of society, may have a "practical" application—to pigeon-hole individuals so that they are even less likely to break out of the sterotype and challenge their powerless role. "The concept of institutional or structural discrimination is becoming more important as it becomes apparent that much inequality results from the policies and procedures of key institutions in our society . . . rather than from consciously biased actions of prejudiced individuals. Indeed, institutional discrimination may well be the primary link between personal ideology and these group inequalities" (Palmore and Manton, 1973).

The government has been allocating resources for a population over 65 who has been cut off from the job market and excluded from central economic and social interactions. A society that forceably retires still productive members, but fails to replace this role loss with meaningful alternatives, is bound to be inefficient in the long run. For this (if for no other) reason, social planners and human-resource specialists should feel compelled to determine (a) what societal pressures operate on groups necessitating their removal from mainstream society and (b) what alternative roles are available both for the institutionalized aging ready for discharge and for the declining community aging. The answer would clearly seem to be to provide preventive and supportive community services enabling the aging to survive in the community even when some degree of assistance for physical, psychological, or social problems is required.

Chapter 3

NORMAL AGING

DEFINING NORMALCY

In order to determine the appropriateness of intervention with an aging client, it is important to differentiate between changes related to normal aging and those that result from pathological processes. Because it had been thought, for example, that loss of teeth was a normal occurrence for the aging person (when it is actually due to gum disease), it was likely that little or no attention would be paid to this phenomenon and the condition would go untreated. Accordingly, an aging client with gum disease (which could be symptomatic of treatable conditions such as nutritional deficiency or infection) would suffer from neglect, called by Butler and Lewis (1973) the "major treatment technique" for the aging. In contrast, obvious physical changes do occur in normal aging, such as greying and loss of hair, and are not to be confused with disease processes, such as gum disease leading to loss of teeth.

Stereotyped expectations about the aging operate in misdiagnosis as well. Some of what is manifested as mental illness, for example, may be due to undiagnosed physical illness. The aging person is frequently misdiagnosed as "senile" when in fact senility is not an inevitable consequence of normal aging. A 46-year-old suffering from hardening of the arteries is diagnosed as arteriosclerotic, but a 62-year-old with the same symptoms is diagnosed as "senile." A 30-year-old suffering from an acute confusional state is comprehensively tested and treated for what is found to be a primary vitamin deficiency, but no tests are ordered for the confused 75-year-old with the same symptoms because this person is instead presumed to be "senile."

In discussing the process of labeling and its effect on clinical judgment, it is necessary to consider the issue of deviance. For example, illness may be defined as behavior that deviates significantly from the norm, making it difficult and impossible for the individual to function within the accepted framework of society, and thus deviant. Or deviance and normalcy may be conceptualized as falling along a continuum of behavior, where deviance would refer to extreme illness and normalcy would refer to absence of illness. A societal reaction theory of illness (Merton, 1957; Gove, 1970; Orcutt, 1973) operates on the premise that cumulative stress may cause an individual to produce nonnormative responses, leading to negative labeling, to future similar responses, and finally to the social identity of an ill person. The production of similar future responses occurs because the persons now labeled as deviant have increasingly limited opportunities in which to exhibit normal behavior, because at this point they are excluded from mainstream society. It has been suggested that environmental stress may lead to the initiation of treatment rather than to illness itself (Mechanic, 1969). In other words, the likelihood that the individual would be labeled as ill may depend on environmental or contextual conditions that are external to the individual, such as the expectations of health professionals and paraprofessionals (Scheff, 1967; Rosenhan, 1975).

Sexuality: A Case in Point

Sexuality, a topic replete with myths about aging, provides a timely subject for examination of the deviance question and presents an excellent example of the interactions of normal social, physical, and psychological aging processes. Problems related to sexuality in the later years of life are bound to trouble old and young at some time in their lives. Sexuality in aging has until recently been a neglected, and even a taboo, topic among health professionals. In fact, even the aging themselves have tended to neglect it, largely in response to the lack of societal interest in the aging as "sexual beings."

It is true that aging may change the ways and means of expressing sexuality, but this is due more to social than physical or psychological constraint. For the aging woman, the expression of sexuality becomes even more critical, as there are four times the number of single older women as men (Harris, 1975). This imbalance is made even more striking by the tendency of some older men to pair off with younger women. For example, it is socially acceptable for a 70-year-old man to go out with a 35-year-old woman, but not for a 70-year-old woman to go out with a 35-year-old man. Consequently, many divorced and widowed aging women have little choice in available partners.

A second social factor that discourages the expression of sexuality involves disapproving attitudes toward sex between consenting aging partners. This is less due to puritanical attitudes toward sex than to the fact that negative stereotypes of the aging are suggestive of inadequacy, lack of vigor, and illness, leading to poor self-image for the aging person. Disapproving attitudes are frequently also found among the families and friends of aging persons, who ridicule them for behaving like "spring chickens." Aging persons who themselves have guilt feelings about their sexuality may use growing older as an excuse not to be sexually active. A third reason that sexuality has for so long remained a controversial topic is the misconception that sexuality implies only physical sex. Sexuality is more a state of mind, and while sexual behavior may be one expression of sexuality, it is not necessarily the central issue. Nonphysical components of sexuality that are particularly important for the lonely, isolated aging person are feeling good about one's appearance, feeling wanted and needed, being able to show affection, and being able to communicate.

Health professionals and paraprofessionals often harbor misconceptions concerning sexuality, sexual potency, and other myths that have grown up about aging and sexuality. One prevalent myth is that sexual potency lessens with age. Research (Pfeiffer and Davis, 1972) suggests that sexual interests and energy are most likely to be maintained in later life by those individuals who were also sexually active in their youth and middle years. Other prevalent myths concern impotence among males and personality changes among females. Healthy males are no more likely to be impotent than healthy females are to succumb to depression. Worry concerning performance may create a self-fulfilling prophesy; while aging males may require more time to achieve an erection, they also tend to maintain it longer. Women may become more sexually active following menopause, possibly because fears of pregnancy have been removed. A prostectomy or hysterectomy need not make any noticeable difference in sexual functioning. In other words, disuse leads to disinterest, which in turn suppresses sexuality, and this is true for normal men and women of all ages. Changes do occur with age (Busse and Pfeiffer, 1969) but in normal persons these decrements in sexual responsiveness need not inhibit normal sexual activity.

It is a serious matter when normal expressions of sexuality are treated as abnormal by health professionals. Consider the frustration of a couple who become interested in one another in a nursing home and cannot even find a closet in which to exchange affection without being on public display, chuckled at by staff as cute, and subject to reprimand by family and friends. This seemingly normal situation may be misinterpreted by others as an abnormal situation because it takes place in an abnormal environment. In other words, determining whether or not the expression of sexuality is appropriate requires consideration of the behavior and context in which it occurs. For example, it would be clearly inappropriate for a person to masturbate in a public setting but not inappropriate to do so in private. Thus, to record on a client's chart that masturbation is a problem, when the person is interrupted doing this at one o'clock in the morning in his or her own room, would be a serious misrepresentation of the facts. On the other hand, sexual acting-out behaviors such as public masturbation may be seen fairly regularly in institutional settings, and would be considered inappropriate even in that context.

Another situation that may be misinterpreted is the demonstration of affection by same-gender persons toward one another. More likely than not, hand-holding between two female patients signals physical affection, not homosexuality. Or a male patient might "come-on" to a female staff member. This situation requires tact and sensitivity; acting flattered by the advance while simply explaining that the attention cannot be returned might be one appropriate response. Health paraprofessionals can be effective in providing correct information and feedback about sexual activities with the goal of reassuring aging persons that expression of sexuality is healthy, normal, and indeed possible at any age.

NORMAL PHYSICAL AGING

In order to understand what happens to people as they age, researchers have developed biological theories of aging, such as the "clock theory," "spontaneous mutation theory," "immunological theory," "enzyme theory," and "protein theory." The clock theory states that aging is inevitably preprogrammed into the developmental sequence from birth; the spontaneous mutation theory states that cumulative alterations in body cells lead to eventual degenerative processes; the immunological theory states that the immune system gradually ceases to function efficiently, causing antibodies to attack normal cells instead of invading microorganisms (Vazquez and Makinodan, 1972); the enzyme theory states that increases in monoaminoxidase, involved in nerve-impulse transmission in the cerebral cortex, cause the hypothalamus to send inaccurate signals to the endocrine system; the protein theory states that protein synthesis, particularly in the RNA messenger protein, becomes less accurate, causing a breakdown in communication among the brain centers. It may well be the case that all of these mechanisms are involved in some extent in normal aging.

The presence of normal physical change with aging, however minute or gradual it may be, can heighten susceptibility to disease. One major threat to physical health in senescence originates from a decrease in the efficiency of overall body homeostasis (Weg, 1973), reflected by the nervous system's decreased ability with age to integrate simultaneously occurring changes in biochemical, muscular, glandular, and circulatory systems. Notably, a slowing in the body's capacity to return to equilibrium following a stressful event is one striking difference between the youthful and the aging individual (Selye, 1970). This slowing may relate to changes on the cellular level, where regenerative capacity slows and there are fewer immunoglobin concentrations (Buckley and Dorsey, 1970). Immunoglobins are products of the body cells largely responsible for producing immunity to disease, and accompanying decreases in antibody activity weaken defenses against disease. These cellular changes have lent support to the immunological theory of aging.

Secondary vitamin deficiencies, frequently involving B12 and folic acid, also contribute to the aging person's heightened susceptibility to disease. Caloric requirements are reduced, due to decrease with age in lean body mass and basal metabolic rate (Exton-Smith, 1974). Decreases occur in secretion of digestive juices, peristalsis, and gastric and intestinal absorption. These normal changes with age affect the uptake and utilization of nutriments.

It is widely accepted that sensory changes with age involve all of the five senses. These normal age-related losses are critical factors affecting the aging individual (perhaps more than any other physical change, since it is through the media of sight, hearing, taste, smell, touch, and proprioception that individuals communicate and receive confirmation of their existence). Decrements in the visual and auditory senses are most pronounced. Visual changes occur along the dimensions of depth perception, color saturation, and visual acuity. Photophobia is more likely to occur, and at the same time the amount of light needed by the aging person to see is three times greater (Crouch, 1967).

Auditory changes, particularly at high frequencies, are more prevalent for males than females (Eisdorfer and Wilkie, 1972). Presbycusis, the term for loss of auditory acuity with age, is characterized by general muffling of sound, making parts of words unintelligible. Although the greatest decrements occur in vision and hearing, other sensory changes that occur with normal aging are impairment of balance and decreased sensitivity to odor, vibration, taste, and temperature.

NORMAL COGNITIVE AGING

As is the case with physical aging, some degree of cognitive decline may be expected in the normal aging process. Mental functioning, or cognition, is affected by the general state of health of the cells and structures of the brain. It cannot be too strongly stressed that there are no psychophysiological changes due to age alone that produce widespread aberrant behavioral responses. For example, changes in the electrical activity in the brain measured by electroencephalogram (EEG) recordings were once thought to be associated with intellectual deterioration, yet recent research reveals that no EEG correlates of cognitive functioning exist in normal community aging populations (Thompson and Marsh, 1973). A word about neuronal loss is appropriate here. Very little neuronal loss occurs after maturity is attained (Brody, 1970); further, neuronal deterioration does not exclude the possibility for adequate compensation (Jarvik and Cohen, 1973).

According to tests of cognitive ability, it had once been thought (Wechsler, 1958) that measurable intellectual abilities peak in early adulthood and then progressively decline. It is now generally accepted that no significant decrease in intellectual ability occurs with advancing age (Shaie, 1974), and where intellectual decline does occur, it is viewed by gerontologists as "attributed to poor environmental conditions for the acquisition and maintenance of intellectual behaviors" (Hoyer, Labouvie, and Baltes, 1973).

When standard tests of cognitive ability are administered to the aging person, interpretation should be made with caution. These tests have for the most part been standardized on populations whose characteristics and requirements in the testing situation differ from those of the aging population (Jarvik and Cohen, 1973). For example, performance deficits rather than cognitive deficits may account for poor tests results (Hoyer, Labouvie, and Baltes, 1973). Factors that may affect test performance are lack of familiarity with testing situation, sensory impairment particularly in the visual and auditory realms, and meaningfulness or relevance of the stimulus material (Arenberg, 1973).

Tests of cognitive ability tend to rely heavily upon the memory component. While aging persons have been found to omit more items than younger persons, they make approximately the same number of actual errors (Eisdorfer, Nowlin, and Wilkie, 1970). There is some slowing in learning new information, but with practice aging persons show the same abilities as younger persons.

Aging persons also tend to recall events that happened in the far past better than they recall recent events, which may suggest that memory decrements with the normal aging may occur in short-term but not in long-term memory. Forgetting that does occur may be explained quite convincingly as the result of social isolation or even of choice: As Cicero said some 2000 years ago, "Old people remember what interests them . . . besides, I never heard of an old man forgetting where he buried his money."

There are no set patterns for cognitive change in normal aging persons (Wang, Obrist, and Busse, 1974), so expectations of cognitive performance must be based on the aging person's individual characteristics rather than on age alone (Birren, 1964).

Mental slowing that does occur as a natural consequence of age does not mean that the individual cannot respond adequately to the environment. Aging persons respond well to perceptual stimuli, despite the apparent comprehensiveness of sensory physical changes, and it must be remembered that decrements represent only a small proportion of the rest of the aging person's functional capacity. Recent research in cognitive processes indicates fairly conclusively that much of what is said about intellectual and cognitive impairment with age is a myth. "The presumed universal decline in adult intelligence is at best a methodological artifact and at worst a popular misunderstanding of the relation between individual development and sociocultural change" (Shaie, 1974).

NORMAL PSYCHOLOGICAL AGING

Physical and cognitive aging are closely linked. When the homeostasis between them is upset, deterioration may appear; so long as homeostasis is maintained in a healthy environment, normal physical and cognitive aging can be compensated for quite readily. The mediating factor in maintaining this balance is psychological well-being.

Normal psychological changes with age may be generally described as "personality" changes. For the most part, these changes are adaptive (Butler and Lewis, 1973) and are complementary to the physical, cognitive, and environmental changes that are occurring simultaneously. Psychological characteristics have in common their involvement with life-cycle completion, such as a desire to leave a legacy, attachment to familiar objects, reminiscing, need for closure. The adjustment reaction ensuing from changes in family or occupational status may erroneously be considered a sign of "mental illness," yet such emotional reactions are perfectly normal considering the serious implications of these age-related crises. Such emotional reactions as depression, anxiety, anger, grief, and guilt are experienced by persons of all ages.

In the aging person, these reactions may be manifested as coping responses, such as selective attention, which would involve forgetting unpleasant events or being hard of hearing only when certain people are about. The particular coping strategy employed by the aging individual will be largely determined by this individual's past pattern of behavior, ability to adapt to change, and "personality" make up. It is difficult to make generalizations about the psychology of aging when individual differences play such an important role in the normal aging process.

While it is true that social, physical, or psychological problems experienced by younger persons may also be experienced by aging persons, the reverse is not necessarily true. There are behaviors that are more likely to typify the older rather than younger person. One of these is the process of the life review, sometimes called "reminiscing," which occurs as aging persons strive to form a cohesive picture of the past. This process is frequently dismissed by health professionals as part of aging pathology, where persons are assumed to have forgotten that they have told a particular story once before or seem to be living in the past. On the contrary, the life review is important to psychological health and should be encouraged. Paraprofessionals working with the aging can be instrumental in helping to "work through" the process of life review by listening with genuine interest and reinforcing past achievements.

In many respects, aging persons have problems very similar to those of younger persons. They have the same needs for dignity, self-esteem, social respect, meaningful occupation, social interaction, and attention. When these needs fail to be met and alternatives are limited, any individual would develop problems of some sort. When younger persons indulge in reminiscing in a therapy situation, it is thought that this bespeaks loneliness, and there is no reason why it should be any less normal for the aging person than it is for the younger lonely person. In other words, there is no need for the diagnosis and treatment process to necessarily proceed differently merely because of the individual's age.

Chapter 4

SPECIAL PHYSICAL PROBLEMS

PHYSICAL ILLNESS

Estimates of the degree of physical illness experienced by the aging need to be interpreted in light of the relative incapacitation these illnesses produce. For example, 86% of aging people are reported to have one or more chronic health problem, yet 81% are still able to get around in the community with no outside assistance (Butler and Lewis, 1973). On the other hand, 52% of retirees (mean age 64.5) sampled in one study (Motley, 1977) had health conditions that precluded or seriously curtailed their ability to work. Where one statistic measures problems due to physical illness in terms of the criterion "ability to get around," another measures it in terms of "inability to work."

It is often the case that problems experienced by the aging person begin developing in middle age and only become evident when the person is older. The early (acute) stage of a problem requires different treatment from the later (chronic) stage. Aging persons with chronic conditions are less likely to be treated successfully than younger persons with the same condition. Thus, the aging person generally has a poorer prognosis because the chronicity of the condition has resulted in multiple pathology, where several different problems exist simultaneously and are interrelated. Once a health problem necessitates intervention, the fortunate aging person who has access to and can afford home health care will be treated by a paraprofessional at the physician's or registered nurse's behest. Visiting physical, occupational, or speech-therapy aides, emergency medical technicians, home health aides, and community volunteers are examples of paraprofessionals who may provide needed services.

Aging persons who cannot remain at home and have no access to alternate services may be admitted to a hospital or health-related facility, for some of the special physical problems outlined below afflict the aging with greater regularity than younger populations. It will not be possible to discuss all the special physical problems encountered with the aging. Paraprofessionals should know that pre-existing conditions are almost certainly involved, and that accumulated pathology plays a large part in the manifestation of any specific disease or deficient state of health.

Nutritional Deficiency

Altered dietary requirements that come as a normal result of the aging process, combined with unmet needs in social, physical, or psychological areas, can create an ideal situation in which nutritional deficiencies may flourish. Appetite is largely dependent upon emotional state; for example, some persons eat more when they are bored or unhappy, and others refuse food under the same circumstances. In other words, food is invested with emotional and cultural meaning, and is not merely a means to an end. Overall, the choice of food is most affected by the aging person's economic status, a choice restricted for most aging persons because of their financial problems. The presence or absence of other persons may also influence eating habits. For example, it may be that eating alone is unfamiliar or that the individual's cooking skills are poor.

Because the senses of taste and smell are less acute with age, food is likely to be less appetizing. This loss of sensory acuity may inhibit the flow of saliva and digestive juices. Poor mouth conditions (e.g., gum infection) may make chewing painful so that certain nutritious foods, such as raw vegetables, are avoided. Even under ideal psychosocial conditions, impairment of the appetite may be enough to discourage the aging individual from eating regular meals. The lowered caloric requirement with normal aging means that second helpings and frequent snacking may result in conditions of overweight and lax body tone. Calcium is particularly important in the aging diet because of the tendency among the aging to develop osteoporosis (softening of the bones), making injury more likely. An additional problem may involve the tendency for some aging persons to suffer from constipation, which may result from the combined effects of lack of exercise, slowing of the rate of absorption of various nutrients, or inadequate fluid intake. The discomfort of the constipated state may act as a further deterrent to normal dietary habits.

More often than not, nutritional deficiencies exist but fail to be diagnosed because they lack specific or observable symptoms (Judge, 1974). An individual in this condition suffers from *subclinical nutritional deficiency*. Were such a person exposed to a stressful situation, the onset of an overt nutritional deficiency could be precipitated. Some primary nutritional deficiencies are straightforward, as with vitamin C deficiency (causing scurvy), thiamine deficiency (causing beri-beri), or vitamin D deficiency (causing malabsorption syndrome). Others are more complex, as with stress-vitamin-C deficiency (causing slowed recovery from illness). This type of a secondary nutritional deficiency, particularly of vitamin B_{12} (Whanger and Wang, 1974), is common in one form or another among most aging individuals.

Special diets for physical conditions such as diabetes, cardiac conditions, obesity, phlebitis, or iron-deficient anemia may require that salt or sugar be removed from food. Prohibited substances (such as sugar for the diabetic person) may be present in unexpected foods and liquids, such as in alcohol or fruit. When the aging person lives in an institutional environment, control can be exerted over the dietary regime; however, when the aging person lives at home and perhaps alone, little control is possible. Here is where a paraprofessional could be of help. The aging person should receive education in nutrition and its importance for continuing good health, and in vitamin supplementation of the diet. For example, some vitamins, such as vitamin C, are merely excreted in the urine when the body has taken in adequate amounts. Other vitamins, such as vitamin E, are stored and do not have established minimal daily requirements. Additional means of safeguarding the observation of a special diet that can be suggested by the paraprofessional is asking the aging individual to keep a chart of the foods eaten, so that a record exists for the professional to look at during the regular check-up. Keeping a chart will also help the individual to see where slip-ups have occurred, and makes it more likely that adherence to the diet will be observed.

Sensory Impairment

Impairment of the sight due to a deteriorative condition such as glaucoma or cataracts can be surgically corrected (and it should be noted that periodic testing for glaucoma can prevent serious degeneration in 86% of the cases [Butler, 1975]). Legal blindness, where eyesight deteriorates past the point of visual acuity, requiring corrective lenses, can be compensated for. However incapacitating it may be, even congenital blindness (from birth) or blindness from trauma need not result in total impairment of the individual's functional capacity. The blind person is not ill, only handicapped, and should accordingly be treated as a normal healthy person. Persons who are blind or who are in the process of losing their sight develop heightened other senses, such as hearing and touch, and as a result may be hypersensitive to their environment. Accurate descriptions of the environment provide blind persons with the tools they need in order to remain oriented. Paraprofessionals can assist the blind person in providing details on shape, texture, and color. The blind person will use tactile exploration, for example, to help in compensating for loss of sight.

Paraprofessionals can also assist the blind person in learning to read by obtaining cassettes of reading material ("talking books"). An increasingly wide range of services for the blind, such as automated Braille utilities, are being provided so that it is not outside the range of possibility for blind aging persons to live and work in the community.

Hearing impairment results in significant hearing loss in over 29% of aging persons (U.S. National Health Survey, 1964), and is the most common of all sensory impairments. It can occur congenitally, gradually, or traumatically. It might involve loss of auditory acuity in only high frequencies (making female voices less distinguishable, for example). Deafness caused by infection can be cured if the onset is recent. Hearing aids can amplify sound enough so that even an almost totally deaf person can still hear vibrations. Paraprofessionals working with the deaf should enunciate clearly and exaggerate the shape of words so that lip reading is possible. Sign language is not difficult to learn and will greatly facilitate communication with the totally deaf who have learned to sign. It should be recognized that many congenitally deaf persons have had to learn to talk in the absence of sound, making their words sound differently, so understanding such persons might be difficult. Deaf persons may speak overly loudly or softly, and would benefit from assistance in modifying sounds to meet normal standards.

Speech impairment taking the form of complete nonspeech may mean that the nonspeaking person may also be deaf and never have been taught to speak. Nonspeech may otherwise result from lack of vocal cords, or the inability to use the vocal cords (as with the person who has undergone an open tracheotomy). It is possible to teach a nonspeaking and deaf person to speak, but it is a difficult procedure, requiring a speech therapist's professional abilities. Persons who have had tracheotomies and relearn speech may sound hoarse and be difficult to understand. Persons who have had laryngectomies can use an amplifier held against the throat, which picks up vibrations that are heard as sounds. Communication using any sounds must be encouraged; some persons may speak in a whisper or refuse to speak by choice. Aging persons with ill-fitting dentures or no teeth will be difficult to understand, as will institutionalized persons who suffer from buccodyskinesia. Paraprofessionals can work effectively with such persons toward regaining normal speech by reinforcing and encouraging all efforts at verbal communication, and by proceeding with patience and understanding.

The following case history illustrates the impact for the aging of real or anticipated sensory deficits on psychological well-being.

> Ms. C., a 63-year-old widow in excellent health, underwent a bilateral radical mastectomy with an uneventful recovery. There was no evidence of lowered self-esteem or depression, and she returned to her active life, which included a full-time job as librarian. Two years later she had a cataract operation, which was only partially successful (i.e., though there was no substantial improvement in her vision she was still not seriously impaired). Recovery from this operation took a year, in marked contrast to her rapid recovery from the cancer operation, and she continued to wear the eye patch long after it was medically necessary. She bitterly complained that she was losing her eyesight, the operation was a failure, she was misled by others about its being a routine operation. She then abruptly retired from work. At home all day, she became obsessed with throwing out furniture, setting her will in order, arranging for a burial plot; she would also talk to herself, forget where she put things, and reminisce about her father. Upon interview, she recognized that she was "sometimes depressed," but felt that therapeutic intervention was for the weak of character or the insane. She blamed her troubles on her unhappy marriage, and felt that she was unappreciated.

One possible interpretation of this woman's gradual decline might be that she denied the anxiety engendered by her cancer operation. However, an alternate explanation should not be excluded, since the mastectomy may have posed far less of a threat to her than losing even a portion of her sight. This reaction is understandable in light of her past livelihood and her self-reliant character. She was, perhaps for the first time, struggling to deal with the fact of her retirement anxiety, social isolation, and possible loss of independence: her aging. Cultural and personality factors make it difficult for this woman to seek or accept intervention. Under the guise of community services, such as companionship therapy or home visitors, needed intervention might be made available; paraprofessionals in such organizations, intervening before this woman becomes more depressed, could provide assistance to her and others of this "hidden" population.

Sexual Dysfunction

Principle and usually interrelated causes of sexual dysfunction among the aging are depression or anxiety, alcohol abuse, fatigue, poor nutrition, or medication effects, yet these are chiefly ignored by the aging as factors. Rather, sexual dysfunction is instead attributed to old age, and continued disuse may then actually result in dysfunction. Unregulated diabetes can result in sexual dysfunction, as will abuse of drugs or effects due to some major antidepressive, tranquilizing, hypertensive medications. By far the major causes of dysfunction are psychological, or relate to sociocultural expectations.

Where it is not physically possible for the aging person to perform, for example in the case of paralysis, paraprofessionals can help the aging person to accept this fact and to rechannel energies in other directions. Even though sexual activity may not be possible, a feeling of sexuality can be reinforced by complimenting on appearance, displaying of verbal affection, and maintaining some appropriate physical contact (e.g., holding hands, giving backrubs). Another way in which paraprofessionals can assist the aging is in facilitating adjustment to situations such as returning home after being hospitalized or institutionalized. While institutionalized, the aging person may have come to feel unattractive and useless. Another physical situation that may affect performance is recovery from surgery or severe cardiac condition where curtailed physical activity has been prescribed. It is important that the aging person's sexual partner be alerted to the possibilities that exist during the aftercare period (such as the inhibiting effects of certain medications) so that the aging person is not made to feel desexualized or impotent.

Bone and Joint Disease

Osteoarthritis is the most common joint disease among the aging, afflicting an estimated 60% (Bierman and Brody, 1976). It may be intermittent and mild or it may take the form of rheumatoid arthritis, which is chronic and in late stages may result in crippling. Deformities can also be aggravated by lack of exercise, poor positioning, or friction over an extended period of time. Special measures must be taken to prevent stiffening in bedridden aging persons afflicted by this problem. Paraprofessionals can assist in providing therapeutic massage with administration of topical preparations to generate heat and increase circulation. Osteoporosis, another skeletal disorder seen often among the aging that results in bone loss and susceptibility to fracture, is four times more common in women than men (Bierman and Brody, 1976). This disease is particularly severe, since it may lead to hip surgery, immobilization, and dependency.

Diabetes

Diabetes mellitus is a condition that affects great numbers of aging persons and may result (in chronic or untreated stages) in physical disabilities such as partial blindness and skin deterioration, or in emotional disabilities such as labile or changeable mood and aggressive behavior. Its role as a cause of aging disability has been seriously underestimated and it has been called the classic example of the aging-versus-disease problem, since "the biochemical changes that occur in apparently mild cases of diabetes may underlie the accelerated development of the disastrous late complications known to be associated with the disease" (Bierman and Brody, 1976). The aging diabetic requires a special diet, and is frequently maintained on medication for this condition requiring daily insulin injections. Paraprofessionals can assist diabetics by making sure that the prescribed dietary regime is closely followed. It may be tempting to get off the regime, because the aging may not attach importance to the consequences of not eating sugar-free foods, not understanding that in uncontrolled stages of diabetes, taking in even small amounts of sugar can precipitate an insulin crisis that can result in convulsions, coma, and possibly death. Continued support for the diabetic client can motivate the individual to form the appropriate dietary habits to ensure continued health.

Stroke

Aging persons undergoing stroke can generally be divided into two categories: (a) those surviving for many years with few attacks, and (b) those having frequent occurrences. Of these, the multiple-stroke syndrome is thought to be closely tied in with hypertension and cardiovascular disease. Aside from paralysis as a result of stroke (hemiplegia, for example), anticipated complications of stroke may include varying degrees of mental disturbance. Stroke, or cerebral infarction, affects more males than females, and may be manifested as one abrupt major stroke or multiple small strokes that are barely noticeable except for gradually decreasing functional capacity. In the case of small infarcts, the individual can learn to compensate fairly well for the disability. For example, where motor functioning in the hand has been affected, the motor cortex of the brain generally retains enough healthy cells to take over, and stroke effects may fade with passing time. A full neurological and physical examination by a professional will be needed to diagnose whether the impairment is temporary or permanent.

Paraprofessionals should look for rehabilitative potential for all stroke clients, particularly in the areas of exercise tolerance and mobility of proximal muscle groups, and overuse of the "good" side in the hemiplegic's case should be avoided. Postural control can be re-established by training the client in such compensatory movements as rhythmical alteration in body sway, supporting reactions of other "working" parts of the body, and righting reactions. Where paralysis has affected the person's ability to care for self, the aging person will undoubtedly become depressed and will require particular attention to motivation.

Where the client has long been confined to a bed or a wheelchair, the idea of leaving the relative security and dependency of the sheltered environment may be frightening and threatening. Paraprofessionals can assist by reassurance and by helping the client look forward to the change. The second step involves retraining muscles, tendons, and nerves that have been in disuse. Important functions of this retraining that can be performed by paraprofessionals involve therapeutic massage. Relearning to walk is a slow, tedious, and frustrating learning task for the client. The individual may become discouraged and want to give up. By being empathetic but firm, and by continually stressing the importance of mobility to the client, the paraprofessional can keep the client on task and assist emotionally in continuing the effort.

Incontinence

Incontinence is a serious physical problem with far-reaching psychosocial implications that affects many institutionalized and some noninstitutionalized persons. The basis for incontinence may be either physical (as in paralysis due to stroke) or psychological (as in severe psychotic depression), and may be urinary, fecal, or of both types. There are different types of urinary incontinence: daytime and nocturnal incontinence, dribbling (or scalding), and stress incontinence (where release of urine occurs in response to stress situations at irregular intervals). It should be pointed out that persons of all ages may suffer from any of these types of incontinence for reason of a medical or even a psychological problem. Causes of incontinence are many: brain damage (loss of cortical control over bladder functions), loss of elasticity of tissues surrounding the urethra, prolapse of urethral mucosa, pressure on the bladder from a tumor or cyst, or infection.

Three methods of dealing with urinary incontinence that have been partially successful (Atthowe, 1972; Brocklehurst, 1974) can be implemented by paraprofessionals. One involves pelvic floor exercises, to raise the bladder roof and remove pressure on the bladder sphinctor, and the other involves the use of pads and appliances for nocturnal incontinence. Finally, bedridden aging persons should be enabled to relieve the bladder of urine (voiding) at regular intervals, and ambulatory persons should have easy access to the toilet. It also helps for the client to be on a controlled amount of liquid and a regular dietary schedule. For example, an aging woman in a nursing home was incontinent of urine and received negative staff attention as a result. She had a miraculous cure for her problems thanks to a health aide's observation that she was drinking large amounts of water (due to an undiagnosed diabetic condition) and was additionally unable to get to the toilet in time because (a) she walked slowly and painfully due to an arthritic condition, and (b) her room was located far from the toilet. Restricting the fluid intake, stabilizing her diabetic condition, and moving her next door to the toilet took care of her problem.

Cardiac Disease

Cardiac disease is the most prevalent cause of death among the aging (and nonaging alike), accounting for 47% of deaths (Siegel, 1972). Of the four basic types of cardiac disease (pulmonary, valvular, hypertensive, ischemic), mixed ischemic and hypertensive are the most common, with ischemic affecting males and hypertension affecting females to a greater extent (Kennedy, 1974). Occurring almost exclusively in the over-65 age group, cardiac amyloidosis, degenerative calcific valve disease, and others often go untreated due to the difficulty in making these diagnoses. It used to be thought that persons with cardiac disease needed to restrict their mobility, including sex. In fact, the cardiac expenditure on the average during intercourse is equivalent to climbing two flights of stairs (Rubin, 1965; Hellenstein, 1971). The heart is a muscle and like any other muscle it needs exercise in order to remain healthy. This doesn't mean overexertion, which is not recommended for anyone, but it does mean that prudent exercise is likely to help retard death from heart disease.

Respiratory Disease

Respiratory disease takes many forms, and while the course of a respiratory illness is long and not necessarily fatal, it is severely incapacitating. Included are chronic bronchitis, emphysema, bronchial carcinoma (lung cancer), and chronic bronchial asthma. Of these, chronic bronchitis is perhaps the most difficult to treat successfully. The etiology of respiratory disease is largely a combination of environmental factors including relative humidity, population density, sunlight, particular composition of the air (pollution), type of occupation, nutrition, and last but not least, cigarette smoking. Even psychological factors may enter the picture, as with intermittent asthma, which is a known psychosomatic stress response triggered by certain stimulus situations (Dekker and Groen, 1956).

Cancer

Perhaps more than any other disease, cancer is feared by the aging because it has become symbolic of death, yet it accounts for fewer deaths than cardiac disease at age 65. Some types of cancer are more prevalent among the aging, especially those relating to the endocrine system (breast cancer in females, cancer of the prostate in males), the large intestine, and the lymph system. Bronchial carcinoma occurs more frequently among the aging, possibly because of accumulated stress factors. Early screening enables treatment to cut down drastically on death due to breast cancer, but intestinal cancer is usually discovered late and surgical removal may result in colostomy, which requires careful post-surgical attention. Cancer is perhaps most feared due to its unpredictable nature; it may run a rapid course or may incapacitate the person for years. Cancer therapies are still controversial and are fairly debilitating in and of themselves, such as chemotherapy. Paraprofessionals can do much for the person suffering from cancer by helping the individual to acknowledge the reality of the disease and by being emotionally supportive to the client and the client's family.

Thyroid Disease

Thyroid disease has received a great deal of attention in aging because it frequently manifests itself as hypothyroidism, presenting a clinical picture similar to an acute confusional state. It is often misdiagnosed as a psychological problem for this reason. Malfunction of this gland causes unique problems in the aging: while the young patient appears agitated, the older patient appears apathetic (Bierman and Brody, 1976). Aging persons with thyroid disease respond differently to common medication than young persons with the same disease, or than nonaffected persons.

MEDICATION

Physical problems are treatable primarily through the combined effects of rehabilitation and medication. While health paraprofessionals will not be administering medication, it is likely that they will be in contact with aging persons who are receiving at least one medication for some physical condition. This is not necessarily because aging persons tend to be "sicker" than any other age group, but because when the aging person becomes ill, it is likely that more than one special problem will appear. As a result of this multiple pathology, drug therapy becomes complicated and it may be part of the paraprofessional's role to monitor the aging person's behavior to observe medication effects.

In adddition to polypharmacy, overmedication has proven a serious problem for the aging, for the reason that aging persons react differently than some younger persons to the same medication and same dosage by reason of their altered metabolism with normal aging. Unfortunately, an alternate explanation could be misuse of medication in order to facilitate "patient management." For the noninstitutionalized aging person who has had medication prescribed, there is the problem of unfilled prescriptions, forgotten medications, self-prescribed remedies, failure to obtain aftercare and regular checkups, and not attaching enough importance to the medication regime. For many individuals, merely getting to the physician or dentist is a realistic problem of large proportion, as transportation may not be available and the cost of medical care may be prohibitive.

Drug side effects are defined as consequences, other than the one for which a drug is used, that result from prescribed medication. This is particularly true with regard to adverse effects involving the individual's physical or psychological state. For example, a common short-term side effect of diuretics (the drug treatment for kidney disease) is edema, swelling of body tissues due to retention of fluids; another example is toxicity in cardiac clients as a result of digoxin. A common long-term effect, produced by maintenance drugs administered daily to the client for a period of several years, that is particularly likely to be seen in institutionalized aging persons is tardive dyskinesia, or pseudo-parkinsonism. This syndrome may be a result of psychotropic medication, particularly in the drug class of phenothiazines, producing a motoric impairment that is irreversible in advanced stages. Symptoms of this disorder may be tremors (particularly of the facial area) rigid or stiff gait, mask-like expression, and muscle tics. Long-term side effects of corticosteroids, the drug treatment for respiratory disease, are brittle bones and failing eyesight.

The list of such side effects is extensive, but one point is important to note. The side effect is frequently misinterpreted as being another disease altogether, or a new cluster of symptoms, and the client is then given an additional drug to reduce these symptoms. In cases of psychotropic medications that are likely to have short-term side effects, an additional drug may be given to reduce the side effect (called a drug interaction) and will itself produce side effects. For example, when pseudo-parkinsonism does occur during the course of psychotropic drug therapy, this side effect will probably be treated with an anticholinergic drug, which in turn can produce a serious drug-interaction effect of cardiovascular embarrassment (CVE).

Drug toxicity can be one of the major causes of decreased mental functioning in the aging. It is extremely important that the paraprofessional, as a member of the treatment team, be aware of this fact and move toward prevention of long-term side effects through careful monitoring of the aging client's behavior.

Chapter 5

SPECIAL PSYCHOLOGICAL PROBLEMS

INTERACTION OF MENTAL
AND EMOTIONAL DEFICITS

For the purpose of discussing psychological problems arising with aging, there are two interacting categories into which these types of problems may be divided. Mental disturbances, the first category of problems, resemble physical disturbances in the sense that they are characterized by observable physical symptoms, have some definite organic involvement affecting the cerebral cortex, and result in impaired physical functioning. Mental disturbances also impair psychological functioning and result in unusual or abnormal behavior, hence their inclusion here. For example, memory deficit resulting from cognitive impairment, a mental disturbance, may be less of a problem than the emotional response to it on the part of the aging (Wang, 1973).

Emotional disturbances, the second category of problems, reflect a more narrow range of problems than those experienced by younger persons (Pfeiffer and Busse, 1973) in the sense that disorders of earlier age tend to include problems in adjusting to general social situations or in developing general coping strategies. Problems in "coping" are no less severe with age, but they tend to be more situation specific (Fiske, 1976). It has been suggested (Wang, 1973) that failure of the aging to adapt to changes in life situations specific to old age, such as change in physical health status for example, may be due less to general socioenvironmental factors (such as stress) than to inadequate coping abilities in response to specific stress-producing situations. Inability to cope with stressful life events may also involve the inability to compensate for deficits, (Foley, 1972; Jarvick and Cohen, 1973) and result in maladaptive behavioral responses. For example, a maladaptive response to sensory impairment in the realm of vision might be severe curtailment of social activities, leading to the development of psychological problems related to isolation, such as depression.

More generally, a "disuse" theory of psychological impairment that links physiological and socioenvironmental factors is suggested by one study (Butler, Dastur, and Perlin, 1965) in which aging persons manifesting "senile" behaviors were found to have no greater metabolic or arteriosclerotic problems than a comparison group of normal community aging. The authors conclude that "the possibility of a 'functional senility,' which could be explained on the basis of disuse or extinction of intellectual abilities, possibly mediated by social adversity and isolation, would be compatible with the findings." The lack of opportunity to practice and maintain intellectual behaviors (Hoyer, Labouvie, and Baltes, 1973) increases the likelihood that understimulation and disuse will lead to psychological deficits in some persons (such as the chronically institutionalized aging).

MENTAL DISTURBANCES

Organic brain syndrome (Dementia) is a diagnosis that applies to any disorder associated with impairment of brain-tissue function. Wide variation in the symptoms of organic brain syndrome is not unusual, and diagnosis is difficult because the syndrome is easily influenced by and confused with other physical (Haase, 1971; Libow, 1973; Settin, 1978) or psychological but nonorganic (Foley, 1972) disturbances the aging person may also have. In addition, none of the symptoms are necessarily restricted to organic brain syndrome alone. To contribute to this confusion, the symptoms are usually discussed in terms of (1) the extent of the mental disturbance (mild, moderate, severe), and (2) the reversibility of the disturbance (acute—reversible, or chronic—irreversible). Characteristic symptoms of organic brain syndrome include (a) disorientation of time, place, name, etc.; (b) impairment of cognitive (intellectual) functioning in areas of problem solving, learning, memory. comprehension, and judgment; (c) emotional lability; and (d) confusion.

When the organic brain syndrome is of an acute (potentially reversible) nature, it would be more descriptive to refer to it as an "acute confusional state." This condition generally occurs as a result of a toxic or ischemic reaction and is reversible when the toxicity is eliminated or the metabolic functioning to the cerebral cortex is restored. Other causes of the acute confusional state could be a severe and specific type of nutritional deficiency, particularly vitamin B_{12} or folic acid (Wang, 1973), trauma or a severe blow to the head, heart disease, drug reaction, and many more. As can be seen, the relationship between physical and mental illness is a close and complex one. Because physical illness is more readily observable, it is more likely that hospitalization, when necessary, will be to medical rather than psychiatric treatment units (Mezey, Hodkinson, and Evans, 1968).

The overlap may be illustrated by the following case history. In this situation, the unnecessarily restrictive treatment for a physical problem (heart failure) led to reactivation of the emotional problem (depression), which in turn led to a mental problem (acute confusional state). Had this client not been correctly diagnosed as having a reversible organic brain syndrome, he might have been relegated to the ranks of the "incurable."

> Mr. T. was a 57-year-old advertising executive who had retired at age 55 and whose expectation was to live only a few more years due to a family history of early death due to cardiovascular disease. As

the months went by he became depressed, slept long hours, obsessively pursued his only hobby, which was working on the car, and became more and more prone to thoughts of suicide. He subsequently admitted himself to a psychiatric hospital, where on formal mental examination he was found to be intellectually unimpaired, but did show signs of severe depression and obsessional anxiety. Following hospitalization and psychotherapy focusing on future planning, he was discharged home to take up jogging, swimming, and gourmet cooking. Two years later he had a mild heart attack, was hospitalized, and upon discharge was prescribed diuretics and a low-salt diet, and was told to also severely curtail his physical activity and stop smoking. Within a few weeks he lost his appetite and became depressed and confused (as a result of the low food intake, low-salt diet, and diuretic therapy, he had developed electrolyte depletion and orthostatic hypotension with an acute confusional state). After being hospitalized for a few days he was again functioning well. He regained his appetite off the low-salt diet, was told to avoid only heavy work, and to cut back (but not necessarily stop) smoking. He then made a slow but lasting recovery, began seeking social contacts, joined a retired businessmen's association, and eventually opened a part-time consulting practice.

The following are examples of organic brain syndrome, or conditions etiologically related to it.

Alzheimer's Disease

Alzheimer's Disease is a progressive deteriorative disease affecting more females than males. Only 4% of all aging persons autopsied in psychiatric facilties were found to suffer from this disease (Busse, 1973), however recent estimates suggest that the percentage for the entire ᵧging population is much higher than is generally believed. Neurological deterioration, involving speech and peripheral motor functions, loss of memory, and thought disorder, characterize the illness. Alzheimer's disease is the closest pathological state to what used to be termed "senility" that has been identified.

Cerebral Arteriosclerosis

Cerebral arteriosclerosis is commonly referred to as hardening of the arteries. This is pathologically different from atherosclerosis, or thickening of the arteries. The condition often exists in all parts of the body, not only in the cerebral cortex. It is important to note that "mental illness" need not complicate the picture. However, when mental illness does accompany cerebral arteriosclerosis, it may result in a clinical picture resembling that of Alzheimer's Disease.

Cerebrovascular Insufficiency

Cerebrovascular insufficiency exists when the metabolic needs of the brain are not met by the existing blood supply. It may be intermittent or continuous and can be due to decreased blood flow (measured by combining the difference in blood pressure between the arteries and the veins with the vascular resistance). Prolonged decreased cerebral blood flow can lead to psychological impairment.

Suggested treatment of organic brain syndrome is controversial. Some current medical treatments being used by professionals with varying degrees of success are: (1) cerebrovascular dilation, either through drug action or carbon dioxide inhalation, (2) hyperbaric oxygenation, using repeated exposure to pure oxygen at 2.5 atmospheres of absolute pressure at 90-minute intervals, (3) metabolic drugs, working on uptake of water, glucose, and oxygen, which supposedly decreases vascular resistance and increases cerebral blood flow, (4) anticoagulants, "thinning" the blood, and rarely (5) therapeutic management, through primarily supportive therapy.

Pseudomentia

Pseudomentia occurs in the case of failure to accurately identify a specific etiological agent responsible for the "demented" state, or in the case of a reversible (e.g., acute confusional) state. Many of the special physical problems outlined in Chapter Four can masquerade as Dementia (e.g., endocrine disorders); another frequently encountered cause of pseudomentia is drug toxicity. The following case history illustrates the caution that must be exercised in diagnosis of mental disturbances and the need to carefully consider the effect of the chosen treatment (in this case, drug therapy) on the aging individual.

> Ms. Y., a quiet 67-year-old widow, lived in a rural setting. She had an unremarkable past history with some mild depression but no psychiatric admissions. She expressed feelings of hopelessness to her daughter who lived nearby, and was urged to visit her family physician who prescribed an antidepressant medication. Several weeks later she became acutely disturbed, frightened, and called her daughter to warn her that the Mafia were after the family and to convince her to go into hiding. She was admitted to a psychiatric hospital on emergency, where she was diagnosed as undergoing a psychotic depressive reaction. Two days later she was fine, and only mildly depressed. Her discharge diagnosis was acute organic brain syndrome with psychosis due to drug intoxication.

No single treatment for organic brain syndrome with the aging exists. The therapy procedures selected for application should take into account such factors as the status of the cerebral cortex itself (severity of organic damage), the presence of other diseases and physical disabilities (multiple pathology), the available facilities (environment), the amount of family involvement (social), the emotional status of the client, and many more interrelated factors. Treatment with this type of client is a challenge, and yet this client is typically ignored and given up for lost, virtually ensuring the fact that the spiral of decline will result in isolation and eventual death from neglect.

Emotional Disturbances

Emotional disturbances are prevalent among the aging as they are with younger persons. However, they are too often ignored in favor of physical problems, are by some incorrectly considered normal to the aging process, and thus are overlooked. For the purposes of treatment with the aging, "neurosis" and "psychosis" will be considered along a continuum of health ranging from normal through abnormal, rather than as separate disease entities.

Anxiety Disorders

Anxiety disorders are extremely common in the aging and are dealt with by the use of defense mechanisms. These are styles of dealing with the world developed by the individual to cope with difficult or anxiety-provoking situations. Defense mechanisms are necessary for normal functioning when used in moderation; it is when the mechanism is overused or used inappropriately that it becomes an emotional problem rather than an adaptive mechanism. The principal defense mechanisms seen with the aging are withdrawal, denial, regression, somatization, and projection. Withdrawal is characterized by social isolation, a general inability to form close personal relationships, hypersensitivity, and seclusiveness. Denial is the refusal to accept reality and ignoring the presence of a problem. Regression involves retreat into earlier, familiar behavior patterns or "childish" behaviors. Somatization is characterized by physical symptoms that are more acceptable than the "real" psychological problem for the client to deal with. Projection is the attribution of unwanted or unacceptable thoughts, behaviors, or feelings to others, when these actually belong to oneself.

Hypochondriasis is often mistaken for somatization. A hypochondriac may either worry excessively about becoming ill, be preoccupied with the body or a part of the body that is believed to be abnormally functioning, or actually manifest symptoms of an illness. Hypochondriasis is one of the most frequently encountered anxiety syndromes with the aging. This reaction may be in part due to the acceptance of the physical "sick role" but fear of "mental illness" in our society. In other words, it is more acceptable to shift anxiety from a threatening psychological area into a more acceptable area involving physical disease. Furthermore, it is rewarding because it insures attention (Martin, 1971). This shift occurs without the individual's conscious awareness in order, perhaps, to get attention or in some cases to "forget" other problems.

A suggested treatment approach for the paraprofessional to take with aging hypochondriacal clients is a firm approach that intentionally does not focus on the physical complaint. This is based upon the theory that a client receiving no attention for complaints and negative statements, while being reinforced for making positive noncomplaining statements, will gradually cease to focus as much on the body. Some of the client's anxiety may then be redirected into healthier, more socially appropriate channels, and the need for attention that often has motivated the expression of hypochondriasis may be addressed directly by providing nonsomatically preoccupied attention.

Affective Disorders

The most prevalent emotional disturbances in aging are affective disorders, which are mood disturbances taking the form of depression usually, or, more infrequently, elation. Although other previously existing diagnostic labels may involve depressive symptomology, such as manic-depressive illness and psychotic depression, they are all primarily expressed as affective disorders with the aging. It should not come as a surprise that affective disorders have been diagnosed in approximately half of the aging outpatient and inpatient population (Pfeiffer and Busse, 1973). Reality-based problems experienced by the aging predispose the aging toward depression. In addition, depression is often a natural reaction to physical illness and may also be attendant upon compensatory responses being made by the body during the process of normal aging.

There are signs of depression that are physical, such as fatigue, weight loss, insomnia, slowing of motor functions, and loss of appetite. And there are signs that are psychological, such as loss of interest in life, social isolation, low self-esteem, pessimism, sadness, apathy, and lethargy. In addition, there may be an anxiety component manifested as trembling, fidgeting or unusually high activity level. No one sign or symptom can be taken as an indicant of depression; rather it is a constellation of many signs and symptoms.

Depression in the aging person is amenable to treatment in a variety of ways, all of them quite effective, particularly when used in conjunction with one another. It is important to take into account the social history of the depressed aging person, since like other emotional disturbances, depression may be closely linked to situational events. Often, when such events are the major precipitating factors in the depression, the depression may go into remission when the situation changes for the better. These emotional disturbances would thus be characterized as adjustment problems, rather than major affective disorders.

The other side of the coin from depression is elation. The client may behave in a "manic" or euphoric manner, be hyperactive, and possibly have short episodes of anger. This disturbance is less outwardly disabling than depression; for example, individuals functioning at a high activity level have been described by staff as "more fun to be with" than a depressed patient. However, its underlying basis is a disturbance of mood just the same. It is possible that elation may be a more adaptive way for the individual to deal with depression, since it ensures continued social contact. This outline of depression has left open for debate the degree to which it may be mediated by or caused by biochemical factors, an issue that is beyond the scope of this discussion.

Schizophrenia

Schizophrenia, the catch-all psychiatric diagnostic category, is not diagnosed as often with the aging client as with younger clients. It is mentioned here because there are untold numbers of aging persons living in institutions who are labeled as schizophrenic and are not any longer schizophrenic. They may have exhibited schizophrenic symptoms at an earlier time in their lives and may now be "burned out." These persons may even be receiving anti-psychotic medication when their symptoms have long ago gone into remission. The effect of a diagnosis stays with a person long after the label ceases to describe the person's behavior. It is a stigma, inevitably coloring the way professionals and paraprofessionsals alike think about the aging, much in the same way ex-convicts are discriminated against even when post-prison records are clearly unblemished for years.

Characterological Problems

Character Disorders, or Personality Disorders, are no more or less frequent among the aging than among their younger counterparts. The difference is one of focus (e.g. the personality variables may be "covered up" by more visible medical problems, or by mild cognitive impairment) or one of definition (e.g. the diagnostician may "forget" to look for these variables). It is less socially acceptable for the aging to have psychological problems than for the younger portion of the population who grew up with therapy as a household word. For many aging, however, a psychological problem means mental illness, stigmatization, possibly incarceration in a mental institution. It is a fearful concept, resulting in an entirely different definition of the word "problem." Alternatively, the conceptual orientation held by the aging toward life may allow for a greater tolerance for discomfort.

Addiction

Among the primary psychological problems of the aging, alcoholism is in the forefront (Gaitz and Baer, 1971). Alcoholism is considered by many an emotional disturbance because it is felt that its origin and behavioral manifestations are psychological. However, some persons are physiologically more susceptible to alcohol addiction than are others. Because it is an addiction, withdrawal results from alcohol deprivation. Thus, the person who is used to a reliable intake of a certain quantity will become irritable, belligerent, hostile, and sometimes suicidal when the intake is cut (as when the individual is hospitalized). Aging persons may begin drinking to take their minds off their problems, which leads to social isolation and depression. It is more likely, however, that the person has a history of heavy drinking, which may escalate due to social-psychological factors. The result of extremely heavy drinking is toxicity due to deterioration of the renal and hepatic systems, and confusion due to massive brain-cell deterioration. In advanced stages it results in a nutritional deficiency of Vitamin B called Korsakoff's syndrome, characterized by loss of memory for recent events, filling in memory gaps by making up false information (confabulation), impaired judgment, and severe disorientation; such persons are otherwise quite sociable and lucid.

Treatment for alcoholism with the aging is similar to treatment for younger persons. It requires, among other things, a strongly supportive environment with intensive building of social support networks. Alcoholics Anonymous has an extremely successful program of intervention for recovering community alcoholics, and can be adapted for institutional use with the aging as well. Nursing homes, for example, do not have bars. Many persons admitted to nursing homes have been used to drinking in varying amounts during their whole lives. Such an abrupt change in a firmly ingrained social, psychological, and even dietary habit has a far-reaching effect, the impact of which is generally not taken into account. Paraprofessionals working with short-term institutionalized clients can provide some of the necessary emotional support to help the aging person to adjust. In community work, the aging person can be urged to seek intervention.

The generalized decline of health that accompanies age has traditionally emphasized the role played by psychosocial losses (Libow, 1973). The search for new predictors of health for the aging (Granick and Patterson, 1971) has brought to light the social-psychological variable "organizational complexity of daily behavior." High complexity, taken together with the absence of chronic cigarette smoking, emerged from among more than 600 medical, physiological, social, and psychological variables as accurate predictors of survival among 65-year-old males. Thus, a behavioral picture characterized by a lack of daily organized, sufficiently complex activities would put an aging man at high risk for mortality. Data such as these have definite implications for psychological intervention.

In the case of aging individuals predisposed toward the development of anxiety and characterologic disorders, psychosocial losses combined with low organizational complexity of daily behavior are likely to serve as precipitants of illness. This is also true with recurrant depressive disorders which are acutely responsive to environmental stress, as in a Dysthymic (Reactive depressive) disorder. Further, "neurotic" disorders which have caused only a mild disruptive influence for the individual during earlier stages of life may, during senescence, be exacerbated by the appearance of major illness, such as an organic brain syndrome. The multiple pathology associated with aging makes diagnosis and treatment of psychological problems an exceedingly complex but always challenging endeavor.

Chapter 6

PARTICIPANT OBSERVATION

Labeling

The participant observer functions as an onlooker, an assessor of behavior within the context of the individual's environment, and a recorder. In so doing, the participant observer, in this case the paraprofessional, cannot be entirely objective for the reasons that (a) the nature of the paraprofessional's role requires some degree of interaction with the person being observed, (b) all observers are influenced by the effect of "set" or expectations upon outcome (for example, one such "set" would derive from theoretical orientation), (c) the classification system for labeling behavior requires the use of institutionalized language, (d) the methodology used in the observation, assessment, and recording of behavior affects the outcome.

The expectations, attitudes, beliefs, and general theoretical underpinnings brought into the observational situation by the paraprofessional will affect the outcome of behavioral observations. For example, the label given to an individual is largely responsible for how this individual will be perceived by others in the future, and how these individuals will view themselves. Labeling behavior is a necessary evil; it is not possible to describe an individual's behavior without resorting to the use of certain technical language that has come into the vocabulary as a means of standardizing (and thus eliminating sources of variation and error) behavior. However, there are times when labeling results in stereotyping, defined as the process of allowing preconceptions to focus on some characteristic of the individual that may prejudice the way that observations are made.

Throughout the literature dealing with definitions of illness, references are made to certain groups of individuals from whom illness is thought to be either more prevalent or more incident. An example of *prevalence* for the group of individuals over the age of 65 would be the greater number of hospital admissions for this sample compared with non-aging samples of persons. Similarly, an example of the *incidence* of illness for the aging would be severity of diagnosis assigned to this one group of individuals that would then be generalized to represent an estimate of the illness for the aging population at large. Such prevalence and incidence measures depend upon the categories into which the sample or population is grouped. This is important in view of the fact that such measures have been extensively utilized as criteria for drawing conclusions about the behavior of aging individuals. Thus, descriptions of persons over the age of 65 based solely upon a descriptive phrase such as "geriatrics," which carries with it a variety of different connotations, should be interpreted with this qualification in mind.

As can be seen, the language used by the participant observer (in this case the health paraprofessional), has critical meaning for the outcome of this aging individual's situation. For example, "since inappropriate behavior is typically behavior that someone does not want and finds extremely troublesome, decisions concerning it tend to be political, in the sense of expressing special interest that can be said to be above the concerns of any particular grouping, as in the case of physical pathology" (Goffman, 1961).

Decisions concerning the health status of a handicapped individual, for example, will largely hinge upon what is meant by the word "inappropriate" used in describing this person's behavior. The word "inappropriate" itself implies a value judgment. While, as was before stated, it is only human to make judgments about others, it should at least be the case that this judge (the participant observer), is aware that these judgments are not made in a vacuum. "Human behavior is viewed as being determined not only by the person's interpersonal ability resulting from previous social learning history, but also by current environmental antecedents and/or consequences of behavior" (Goldfried and Davidson, 1976).

The theoretical orientation of the participant observer is one variable that powerfully affects clinical judgment. For example, a psychodynamic orientation would focus upon the individual's traits or characteristics, whereas a behavioral orientation would place emphasis upon what a person does in various situations. In one study (Langer and Abelson, 1974), the effect of labeling on clinical judgment was experimentally investigated. Psychodynamic and behavioral clinicians viewed a videotaped interview of a stimulus person (actually a job applicant). Clinicians were divided into two groups: the experimental group, in which clinicians were told that the stimulus person was actually a patient, and the control group, in which clinicians were told the person was a job applicant. All clinicians then completed a questionnaire evaluating the stimulus person. Behavioral therapists described the stimulus person as better adjusted than did psychodynamic therapists; experimental group clinicians rated the stimulus person as significantly more disturbed than did control-group clinicians. Thus, therapy orientation strongly influenced clinical judgment. If clinicians were not given the label "patient," they would attribute a very different and less negative set of personal characteristics to that individual.

Perhaps the most widely known demonstration of labeling is a field study (Rosenhan, 1973) in which eight persons who knew the purpose of the study voluntarily checked into a mental institution. They were observed, evaluated, and assigned a diagnosis of schizophrenia based upon the fact that they all reported having auditory hallucinations. This is not the surprising part of the study. Following admission, these eight persons ceased to exhibit any further evidence of unusual, deviant, inappropriate, or hallucinatory behavior. Just the same they continued to be labeled as mentally ill upon review of their cases up to and including their time of discharge. This study vividly demonstrates that the label assigned to an individual (e.g., schizophrenia) more powerfully influences treatment and outcome than does the actual behavior exhibited by the individual.

These two studies demonstrate that diagnosis, which is by necessity a judgmental classification process, is based in large part upon the observer's expectations of behavior. While paraprofessionals do not make diagnoses, they do have expectations that are irrevocably built into the fabric of the observational process. Some expectations are admittedly less desirable than others; it is (a) when expectations take the form of prejudice, a negative stereotype, or (b) an unfavorable bias or attitude toward an individual that particular benefit accrues to examining perceptions of individuals belonging to different status groups, such as the aging.

BEHAVIORAL ASSESSMENT

Behavior observation with the aging requires not only the knowledge of what to look for and how to best describe it, but also a trained eye for the sometimes minute changes in physical or psychological status that could make an important difference. Observations may be made in direct or indirect manner, depending on the feasibility of conducting the observations within the natural setting and the nature of the information required. Direct observation of behavior is felt by behaviorally inclined clinicians to be the most useful of all assessment procedures (Paul, 1969). While using this method, "It is necessary to develop some sort of classification system, so that attention can be drawn to specific aspects of the environment as well as to the individual's response to it"

(Goldfried and Davidson, 1976). In direct assessment, teams of raters (participant observers) who have been trained in behavioral observation procedures might follow and observe the individual. Typically, a finite number of behaviors that have a high probability of occurring are charted at regular intervals for one particular time segment, at which point observations are discontinued until the next time segment is due.

For example, the goal of the participant observer as decided by the treatment team might be to collect information about a client who is wheelchair-confined and thought to have a paralyzed leg, because the individual alledgedly could move his legs as reported by paraprofessional ward personnel. The participant observers proceed by working in pairs, circulating clockwise about the room, and making one full revolution of the ward where the client is located every three minutes. At a fixed interval, occurring at the minute-and-a-half mark, they independently observe the client for 15-second intervals and then make ratings on the charge indicating whether the client had performed any of two target behaviors: (1) movement of the left leg or (2) movement of the right leg. If movement occurs a line is drawn through the box on the chart representing that particular segment of time. Another set of boxes on the chart indicates the context in which the client does or does not perform the target behavior: presence of a staff person in the room or absence of a staff person in the room. At the end of the hour, 20 such observations per participant observer have been made, and at the end of a two-week period observations are tallied and a graph is drawn charting the client's behavior.

This hypothetical example illustrates one method of assessment that can be effectively performed by the paraprofessional in a health setting or a non-health setting. Its advantages as an assessment technique are that (a) it takes into account contextual variables (e.g., effect on staff client's "faking" paralysis), (b) it eliminates the need to use evaluative language, (c) it samples the target behavior over a period of time, insuring that the behavior observed is not merely coincidental, and (d) it enables the participant observer to be unobtrusive after several days (part of the normal ward atmosphere). The purpose of having more than one participant observer is for reliability, which can be calculated by summing the ratings across two or more raters and then dividing by the number of raters.

CLINICAL INTERVIEWING

It may not always be possible to use such direct behavioral-assessment techniques, and in some cases it may not be desirable, given the nature of the behavior in question or given the goal of assessment. When the goal is to elicit information as well as probing and exchanging information with a client, the clinical interview is a more appropriate assessment technique. It can be conducted by a trained paraprofessional so long as the paraprofessional leaves the role of evaluation to the professional. Taking information from an aging individual may involve more than the ordinary amount of skill because of (a) sensory deficits, which may make communication more difficult, (b) the need to establish rapport by building trust and allaying anxiety, and (c) the increased requirement for feedback (Bellucci and Hoyer, 1975).

Interviewing is not only a technique, but an art. The interview has a specific beginning, center, and end. Initial contact with the aging person involves a greeting, to make the person feel comfortable, provide structure, and indicate clearly the goal of the interview (Goldfried and Davidson, 1976). No matter what the theoretical orientation, the interview should incorporate the following empathic characteristics: (a) establishing trust, (b) building rapport, (c) helping the person identify feelings, (d) communicating understanding of the person's feelings, (e) making nonjudgmental reflections, (f) paraphrasing, (g) keeping questions to a minimum, and (h) allowing freedom of expression (Benjamin, 1974). This list of desirable characteristics may sound like a tall order, but it includes things that any involved, caring, helping person does intuitively.

The one element of empathic interaction with an aging person that requires clarification is that of nonjudgmental reflection. Just as a mirror reflects back an image, the interviewer should be able to reflect back what the aging person is trying to communicate, both verbally and nonverbally. For example, when the aging person states, "I just can't stand my neighbor any longer," nonjudgmental reflection might mean responding with, "It sounds like you really can't stand your neighbor." In paraphrasing, the response might be, "You seem to really be fed up with you neighbor." In this manner, the paraprofessional stays within the realm of nonevaluation, while providing a sounding board and eliciting further information.

A second feature of the interview involves gathering information. In information gathering the format is a question-and-answer interplay, and it goes without saying that the situation will be nonproductive if it sounds like an inquisition. Closed questions elicit the least information. For example, to ask the aging person, "Do you feel ill?" leaves closed the possible number of responses the person can give to the question. An open-ended question eliciting more information would be, "Please describe for me how you have been feeling." Open-ended questions begin with the following words: How, when, where, who, why, and what. In the process of conducting the information interview, problem issues may emerge that require definition. Defining issues involves mutual cooperation between the interviewer and the person being interviewed with the goal of establishing concrete specifics, yielding an accurate portrayal of the situation.

The rest of what happens in an interview is very much determined by the personal style of the interviewer. In other words, the paraprofessional will do best by behaving naturally, speaking plain, nontechnical language, in a warm and nonthreatening manner. Again, the key word is nonjudgmental. The main point is not to enter the observational situation with preconceived notions about what will be found. For example, the paraprofessional who is convinced that the client has severe psychological problems will be much more likely to observe symptoms that support this preconception than will the paraprofessional who studiously avoids preconceptions.

Interviewing skills will enhance the effectiveness of the paraprofessional in any setting, and particularly with the aging because of the difficulty in administering standardized tests with the infirm or handicapped aging person. Still, most of what the paraprofessional will be doing will be of an observational nature. Accurate observations may be made during all interactions; it need not be that a formal behavioral assessment or interview situation be in effect. The meaning of the term "participant observation" implies that in the act of interacting with the client, the paraprofessional observes. In fact, the observations may be more meaningful because they will be unplanned and will occur spontaneously in a natural environment. Observations are made about symptoms that are either (a) objective findings that can be seen, felt, or heard by the paraprofessional, (b) subjective findings that can be reported by the aging person, or (c) cardinal findings that can be directly measured by the paraprofessional. Behavior is what is known to exist because it has been observed; it is seen, heard, or even sensed as it happens, but it is not inferred or deduced.

OBSERVATIONAL TECHNIQUES

Many of the problems experienced by the aging person stem from neglect. For example, during an initial interview, the aging person may present the problem of inability to walk due to severe foot pains. Upon examination, the client is found to have a bad callous requiring surgical removal. Had this condition been observed early in onset, at an acute state of development, the chronic condition would not have set in. Had a paraprofessional noted in a chart that this client appeared to be limping or that the client reported foot pain, it is possible that a surgical procedure could have been prevented. Notations in a chart need to be precise, legible, in ink, indicating the time and date of observation and the observer's name. In this manner, the client's profile is always up to date and available to all members of the treatment team.

In the case above, the aging client's objective symptoms would include limping or refusal to wear shoes on the affected foot, a subjective symptom would be the client's complaint of foot pain, and a cardinal symptom would be weight gain due to inactivity. It is important to note that the paraprofessional cannot assume that the client is experiencing foot pain just because limping or weight gain is observed, because this would be an inference made in the absence of objective data. Nor can the paraprofessional assume that limping will necessarily occur just because the client complains of foot pain. In other words, what can be observed and recorded with certainty are the facts that callouses were seen, limping was seen, the client complained of pain, and so on.

Examples of findings that may be observed include the following basic areas of the body, which should be looked at routinely:

(1) Skin—Objective: abnormal redness, scratches, rash, dryness, moistness, temperature, elasticity. Subjective: client complaints of itchiness, pain, sensitivity.

(2) Eyes—Objective: expression, swelling, redness, tearing, discharge, twitching, dark circles under, inability to read. Subjective: client complaints of blurred vision, itchiness, pain, inability to see normally.

(3) Ears—Objective: discharge, swelling, secretion, inability to hear, disequilibrium. Subjective: client complaints of abnormal sensitivity or insensitivity to sound, pain.

(4) Nose—Objective: discharge, swelling, redness, inability to smell. Subjective: client complaints of difficulty in inhaling, stuffiness, abnormalities of smell.

(5) Head and Face—Objective: position, swelling, bruises, spasms or tics, facial expression, condition of scalp. Subjective: client complaints of itchiness, tenderness, stiffness, pain.

(6) Mouth and Gums—Objective: discoloration, bleeding, discharge, sores, odour of breath, missing or decayed teeth, missing inlays, fillings, poor fit of

            dentures, difficulty in chewing, refusal to eat. Subjective: client complaints of tenderness, aching, pain.

(7)   Throat—Objective: hoarseness, swelling, difficulty in talking or swallowing. Subjective: client complaints of soreness, pain.

(8)   Chest—Objective: coughing, wheezing, gasping, expectoration, abnormal respiration, lumps. Subjective: client complaints of not feeling "right", pain, difficulty in drawing deep breaths.

(9)   Abdomen—Objective: swelling, lumps, unusual discoloration, unusual bowel-movement or urine characteristics. Subjective: client complaints of tenderness, difficulty in elimination.

(10)   Extremities—Objective: edema (swelling), deformities, tremor (shaking), varicosities (swollen veins), nail problems, unusual temperature of limbs. Subjective: client complaints of stiffness, weakness, cold, tingling, or numbness.

(11)   Overall Condition—Objective: changes in weight, temperature, appetite, energy level, posture, sleeping behavior. Subjective: client complaints of abnormal thirst, insomnia, fatigue, drowsiness, lack of appetite, dizziness. Cardinal: direct measurements of temperature, pulse, respiration, weight, blood pressure.

Psychological observations are more complex than physical observations for the reason that the symptoms being observed are internal processes. That which occurs within the individual emotionally or in the individual's cerebral cortex cannot be directly observed. What are directly observable are subjective observations involving the aging person's feelings, perceptions, and emotions that the aging person reports directly to the paraprofessional. For example, the aging person reports that white butterflies are flying around outside when the context observed is that it is snowing and there are no butterflies to be observed. The terminology that has evolved to describe the seeing of that which is not there comes easily to mind: "hallucination." However, the paraprofessional has no definite evidence that the client is hallucinating. All that is known is that the client has said that butterflies are outside and this is what the paraprofessional should record on the chart and relate to the professional staff. It may be that knowledge of this particular person enables the paraprofessional to know that this person has an idiosyncratic, a poetic way of speaking about snow (white butterflies), and this is relevant information. It is then the professional's role to interpret and diagnose.

As with physical observations, the psychological behavior of the aging person may be observed at any time. Because behavior is situation-specific, it is desirable to observe the individual in as many contexts as possible. For example, when alone in their room, clients may be talkative, but when interacting with others at a social gathering clients may be seclusive. No behavior is without meaning. For example, an aging client may ask the paraprofessional six times in six minutes for a match to light a cigarette that has already been lit six times; there is some meaning to this behavior, possibly a plea for attention, possibly a severe short-term memory deficit, possibly that the cigarette was never really lit. Despite the range of interpretations that could be made, the fact remains that the observation made by the paraprofessional should be "Mr. T. asked that his cigarette be lit six times in six minutes at 3. p. m. on June 23."

Psychological observations include the following general categories:

(1) Disorientation and Confusion—Objective: inaccurate report of date, time, place, or name. Disorientation may be due to boredom or learned helplessness (being taught to be so dependent that there is no point for the client in remaining oriented). Confusion may be a symptom of mental or emotional disturbances. Subjective: client complaints of not being able to remember things, of being called by the wrong name or age, of missing meals or engagements, of claiming not to know family members.

(2) Suspiciousness—Objective: self-protective and guarded behaviors, eye expression, wariness, belligerence in actions or

speech. Subjective: client complaints of being fearful, taken advantage of, talked about, or plotted against by others. Be careful in judging these suspicions as irrational until it has been established beyond any doubt that the complaint has no basis in truth.

(3) Apathy—Objective: listlessness, loss of appetite, blank facial expression, mumbling speech, sagging posture, slowed reactions to stimuli, dull eye expression. Subjective: client complaints of lack of meaning to life, boredom, not wanting to do anything, feeling tired and lacking energy.

(4) Inappropriate Verbal Behavior—Objective: wandering off topic, talking to self constantly, talking to imagined other persons, disconnected speech, rambling nonsensical speech, hostility, sobbing, yelling or screaming in nonthreatening situations, abusive language. Subjective: client complaints of hearing voices, deafness, speech anxiety (extreme forms of stuttering, inability to talk at all).

(5) Inappropriate Nonverbal Behavior—Objective: bizarre dress, strange postures, stereotyped movements (performing a motion over and over agan), strange facial expressions, self-destructive behaviors, aggressiveness toward other persons without provocation, excessive dependency or antisocial behavior. Subjective: client complaints of being out of one's own body (depersonalization), strange thoughts, bizarre preoccupations or delusions.

Other than objective observations of psychological states made in this manner, there are questionnaire or so-called paper-and-pencil assessment methods for obtaining information of a psychological nature. These subjective assessment devices typically involve filling out a rating scale on the individual's level of functioning, or perhaps administering a standardized questionnaire to the aging person. These tests will be requested by a health professional. Before obtaining any information whatsoever from the individual, the observer must obtain an informed consent; if the individual does not give written informed consent to the testing procedures, the testing cannot be accomplished with that individual.

An example of a self-report inventory used in nursing homes, long-term facilities, and community health centers is the NOSIE-30, a Nurses' Observation Scale for Inpatient Evaluation (Honigfeld and Klett, 1965), a 30-item behavior-rating scale to be completed by staff, ward personnel, paraprofessionals, nurses, or other persons familiar with the individual over a period of at least two days. Each item is rated on a five-point scale and seven-factor scores are derived from the items: social competence, social interest, cooperation, neatness, irritability, manifest psychosis, and psychotic depression. It takes no longer than five minutes to fill out and provides a comprehensive overview of the person's verbal and nonverbal behavior, mood, and psychological status.

Chapter 7

THERAPEUTIC INTERVENTION STRATEGIES

TREATMENT WITH THE NORMAL AGING: DOES AGE REALLY MATTER?

Treatment strategies with the aging largely parallel those applicable with other-aged populations. However, normal aging does result in certain physical and emotional changes, and it is only realistic to design treatments that accomodate these changes. It should be stressed that, despite special age-related changes, the difference in treatment is one of emphasis rather than strategy. For example, the client for whom insight-oriented therapy is appropriate will be determined by the presenting problem rather than the chronological age; the difference might be in the particular topics emphasized during application of the insight-oriented approach.

Changes that necessitate different treatment foci may be categorized into four general areas, corresponding to changes undergone by the aging client as part of normal development: (1) overall decreased efficiency of all body systems (e.g., heightened susceptibility to disease, slowed capacity to return to equilibrium following stress); (2) decreased sensory functioning; (3) adjustment reaction to losses (e.g., depression resulting from death of family or friends, retirement from occupational structure or from accustomed social roles, relocation); (4) impairment in cognitive functioning (e.g., decline in short-term memory, lowered performance on intelligence tests).

Since, from a medical standpoint, even the normal aging person's clinical picture "is dominated by multiple chronic diseases and processes which, by definition, persist once they have appeared and which therefore accumulate in an elderly population" (Ford, 1968), it would be unrealistic to expect that psychotherapy with the aging should not deal with disease and disability of the physical self. With regard to the first area, that of overall decreased efficiency, reality-based therapy directed toward the goal of acceptance of disability would be appropriate. However, this area is the least difficult for the aging to accept; in fact, one problem for many normal aging persons concerns their tendency to age, psychologically, before it is entirely necessary. Part of this is traceable to ingrained attitudes toward aging held by older persons themselves, that, for example, they will become incapacitated due to chronic age-related disease (e.g., arthritis); part is traceable to others' stereotyped attitudes toward aging.

Further, somatic preoccupations may result from the expectation that such illness necessarily accompanies aging to a crippling extent, and from the reinforcement that aging individuals may derive from taking on a "sick role." Liederman, Green, and Liederman (1967) report that complaints of an outpatient group of aging were chiefly somatic, but that clients realized that their aches and pains had a functional overlay. Acknowledgment of the role played by emotional distress in producing symptoms is thus a major therapeutic goal in treatment of the individual with physical complaints of psychogenic origin. For example, clients' ability to understand, for example, that the arthritis only flares up when they are upset, but that they feel fine (even though the arthritic condition may still be there) and can cope effectively when they are engaged in pleasant events, can make the difference between successful adaptation to physical illness and serious psychological impairment.

The second of the areas of normal change, decreased sensory functioning, can be extremely difficult for the aging person. The problem is compounded by the fact that many aging are not fully educated concerning their sensory losses and may be unaware of the normal ability of the sensory system to compensate for such losses. In addition, multiple losses are the rule, and these are much more difficult to deal with than single losses. Thus, in spite of the fact that the aging person gradually undergoes these losses and that they are usually not incapacitating, the aging individual views them with trepidation and fear. They may also be symbolic of impending death, signaled by losing sensory contact with the environment. Reactions to sensory loss can be varied, and may be evidenced as hostility, anger, intense anxiety, or depression.

Hearing loss is more likely to adversely affect psychological functioning than either sight, gustatory, tactile, or kinesthetic sensory loss (Busse, 1967), and has definite implications for treatments utilizing primarily verbal modalities. More than any other group, the deaf and hard-of-hearing are excluded from group therapy because of their alleged inability to engage in normal verbal behavior, or because other group members would have to shout in order to be heard. Proper screening of the aging person suspected of having hearing loss should be conducted so that hearing aides can be provided and lip-reading techniques can be taught.

Because hearing impairments are less obvious than visual impairments, others may remain unaware that the individual is experiencing difficulty with hearing and may instead misinterpret certain behaviors. Aging persons with hearing impairments may feel isolated, frustrated that they cannot hear, suspicious that others talk about them, or left out of conversation on purpose. Due to some persons' inability to monitor their own volume, they may alienate other aging persons by shouting, may interrupt, make irrelevant statements during conversation, or appear confused. It's no wonder that the interaction between hearing loss and depression is well established (Shore, 1976).

Aging persons with sensory losses cannot necessarily expect others to be aware of or sensitive to their impairment. Assertiveness training for such persons emphasizes the need to inform others matter-of-factly and appropriately to take account of the impairment (e.g., "could you speak more distinctly so I can read your lips") and is an important adjunct to therapy. Exploring feelings about sensory loss, such as anxiety about becoming dependent, fear of worsening impairment, embarrassment about appearance, and feeling about the aging process in general, can educate staff as well as clients (Hickey, 1975).

The third area of change occurring with normal aging, that of adjustment reaction to loss, applies at some time or other to all individuals. Regardless of the level of emotional stability of the aging individual, there will be a serious reaction to losses that inevitably remind one of one's own mortality. In dealing with such losses, there is a danger in dismissing aging as a "social disease" that needs only a socially oriented approach to mental-health problems. That is, adjustment problems or personality disorders requiring psychological intervention may be ignored in favor of superficial treatment (e.g., need for increased activity or expansion of network of friends). For problems involving serious emotional losses, "The psychological treatment goal is obtaining insight and restitution possibilities within the limits of the life situation and individual personality. Losses in every aspect of late life compel the elderly to expend enormous amounts of physical and emotional energy in grieving and resolving grief, adapting to the changes that result from loss, and recovering from the stresses inherent in these processes" (Butler and Lewis, 1973). Perhaps the ultimate loss, physical and emotional, is death.

DEATH AND DYING: A CASE IN POINT

Life expectancy has now reached so far beyond the age of 65 that aging no longer needs to carry with it the connotation of death. Yet death and the concept of aging continue to be linked, particularly in the health professions, where decline and deterioration are considered to be synonymous with aging and where death is treated antiseptically (Weisman, 1972). Non-Western cultures, on the other hand, view aging as a natural part of the life cycle, a last developmental stage in a series of stages of growth, a biological reality. Such cultures are more likely to contain extended family structures that decrease alienation from death (as opposed to the nuclear family whose elderly are less likely to live at home until they die). Individuals within extended families containing elderly persons play meaningful roles in the process of death, and become skilled in providing emotional support. Within extended-family systems, religion is more likely to play an integral role in attitudes toward death. For many, release from the physical into the spiritual realm makes death transitional rather than a final stage.

According to Kübler-Ross (1975), there are four stages preceding acceptance through which dying persons pass: denial, anger, bargaining, depression. Denial, a defense mechanism, protects the individual from reality until coping mechanisms are strengthened; anger comes with partial acceptance; bargaining, defined as ambivalence, is characterized by the belief that a reprieve will occur; depression, or preparatory grief, signals acceptance and is often accompanied by reminiscing, life review, and re-energization.

It has been suggested (Kastenbaum and Aisenberg, 1976) that there is better psychological preparedness for death among aging than among younger persons. It may well be that aging persons react in a qualitatively different way to the issue of death. Thus, Kübler-Ross's developmental paradigm may not pertain to aging clients at all, but to other-aged populations, or only those individuals suffering from terminal illness. This directs attention to what may be yet another myth about aging: that for the aging, death is an aversive topic.

Given that death and dying need not necessarily enter the therapeutic picture in terms of self-assigned problems of aging clients, it may be that aversion to death resides in attitudes of health-care providers. For example, the "death anxiety" often attributed by therapists to the aging may more accurately reflect their own anxiety projected onto the client. Research on attitudes of the aging toward death (Jeffers, Nichols, and Eisdorfer, 1961) supports the notion that death is more feared by persons working with the aging than by the aging themselves. A too-frequently expressed opinion is that there is no point in providing in-depth psychiatric treatment, working on discharge plans, or "teaching old dogs new tricks," when one's client is just going to die anyway. This not only reflects ageism in the health professions, but strongly emphasizes the degree to which aging and death are associated.

No two persons have the same personality, attitudes, or experiences, and while there may be commonalities among individuals, no two aging persons will deal with their disability, illness, or impending death in the same manner. Such individual differences have been emphasized by research conducted within psychiatric institutions (Feifel, 1959); examining aging psychiatric residents' perceptions of death, it was demonstrated that "psychotic" residents assigned more violent imagery to their imagined deaths than did nonpsychotic residents. Research without institutions on this topic must take into account such factors as past experience with others' deaths, prior hospitalization, marital status and family responsibilities, and religion, all of which cannot help but influence the way a person feels about death. Perhaps those persons who feel that their lives have been worthwhile may experience less conflict about death than persons whose life satisfaction is low, who feel that they have failed, regret the past, or have seriously unresolved conflicts. On the other hand, it may be that those who suffer from long-term disability or painful illness, or those for whom social isolation is acute may be more easily reconciled to death.

Because few health professionals care to work with aging (not to mention dying) clients, the primary care providers for this neglected and needy population will be the paraprofessionals. In this as in other therapeutic encounters, relationship factors play a major role in the helping process. A task for paraprofessionals within this relationship would be to communicate that emotional reactions (such as anger directed outward toward others or inward toward oneself) are legitimate and acceptable feelings to express. Far from precipitating decline, open discussion of death may come as a relief, particularly if death has been a taboo topic in the family (Feifel, 1963; Wahl, 1973).

PHYSICAL INTERVENTION

Traditionally, because paraprofessionals working with the aging have been employed within institutions, such as nursing homes, therapeutic intervention has been focused on physical problems. The key words in intervention are support, rehabilitation, and self-care: support referring to the capacity of the paraprofessional to act in a positive, helpful manner toward aging clients, rehabilitation referring to the restoration of normal functioning following illness in order to attain self-sufficiency, self-care referring to teaching the aging to help themselves.

Of these, self-care is perhaps the most important key concept for the paraprofessional (Zerbe and Hickey, 1975). While teaching self-care skills may at first take some extra time, the benefits are numerous. In addition to discouraging helplessness and dependency, self-care frees staff to perform other-than-custodial tasks that require expertise. For example, bedridden or multiply handicapped persons may not be capable of implementing techniques to help themselves 100 percent of the time; they must nonetheless be allowed to function independently to the furthest extent of their potential. Other persons, for example those who have been overprotected by staff or family, may be fearful at the prospect of helping themselves after being taken care of for so long and might resist self-care. Paraprofessionals can help such aging persons by explaining how self-care (walking instead of using a wheel-chair) benefits them, rewarding them for implementing self-maintaining behaviors, listening to problems, and offering emotional support where appropriate.

Principal areas of physical intervention that can be implemented entirely by the paraprofessional are movement and exercise, and personal care and hygiene. Paraprofessionals will need to be informed of guidelines to follow, particularly when assisting the aging person in physical intervention procedures: (1) making sure the procedure is prescribed for the client; (2) informing the client of what is about to take place and, if necessary, explaining the procedure; (3) recording what has been done in the client's chart.

Movement is of paramount importance in maintaining health, both for the normal aging in order to prevent illness and for the aging with special physical problems in order to prevent further deterioration and to promote recovery. The area covered by movement involves movements made by the client in bed, ambulation transfers, and physical exercise; it does not include range of motion exercises. Moving a client in bed may be necessary in order to change linens, aid in washing and dressing, and most importantly, to prevent stiffening of joints, shortening of muscles, and decubiti (bed sores). When moving a client, the posture taking while lifting must be comfortable, or there is risk of muscle strain. Typically, feet are separated, one foot is placed ahead of the other for stability, the back is kept straight, and the knees are flexed to take pressure off the back muscles. Clients who are fully or partially confined to bed may be gotten up at least once a day and if possible encouraged to ambulate.

It is important to promote independence by, for example, discouraging excessive use of the wheelchair when the client is capable of using a walker, a cane, or of walking unassisted. Some aging clients, particularly those who have suffered injuries by slipping and falling, may be fearful of walking unassisted; some may enjoy the attention and dependency fostered by the wheelchair and be reluctant to lose it. Aging persons who do not have proper foot attire or who are required to walk on slippery or waxed surfaces will be even less motivated to try. For this reason, it is important to determine the environmental factors that may be affecting decreased motivation.

For the normal aging, exercise is a powerful variable in the prevention of illness; for the infirm aging client, exercise can minimize disability and speed recovery. (Comstock, Mayers, and Folsom, 1969). There are four basic exercises with which paraprofessionals should be familiar: 1) therapeutic massage, 2) passive-motion exercises, 3) isometric exercises, and 4) active-motion calisthenics. In addition, specific parts of the body may be exercised through therapeutic-recreational means such as drawing or music to exercise stiffened fingers. Therapeutic massage is employed to increase circulation, firm muscle tone, maintain skin flexibility, relieve tension or muscle ache, and generally provide some reassuring physical contact. Passive-motion exercises are employed to increase flexibility, specifically in the connective tissue and joints. The aging client should also receive instruction in self-administration of limited passive-motion exercises such as ankle rotation and finger flexion. Isometric exercises are employed to build body tone and muscle strength by the principle of opposing muscle groups in tension and relaxation. Active-motion calisthenics are employed with the healthy aging for physical fitness.

In any type of exercise it is important to carefully assess the aging individual's limitations so that unnatural or discomforting positions are avoided, particularly since joints become less flexible and bones more fragile with age. Specific exercises for areas of the body affected by disease or disability (e.g., paralysed by stroke or spinal injury) need to be designed by a professional, but may be carried out by paraprofessionals. Dance therapy, while also a recreational activity, provides an enjoyable and thoroughly balanced exercise regime (Caplow-Lindher, Harpaz, and Samberg, 1979). Particularly for institutionalized clients (Powell, 1972) a few minutes of yoga or calisthenics can restore suppleness to stiff muscles, limbs, and back (Quilitch, 1974), and produce positive psychological effects; walking a treadmill increases circulation and decreases heart rate and systolic blood pressure (Stamford, 1972).

Personal care is an aspect of intervention that is too often neglected, possibly because of the stereotyped "youth culture" expectation that physical appearance is less important for the aging. This negative stereotype produces the effect of loss of interest in one's sexuality, low self-esteem, and negative self-image. Other persons will react less positively to being with aging clients whose personal care is poor. Aside from these obvious emotional components, poor personal hygiene may lead to disease; for example, failure to attend to dental hygiene or denture care can result in gum disease. When infirm, the aging need more frequent mouth care because they may breathe primarily through the mouth, resulting in drying of mucous membranes and mouth odor as a result. Activities of daily living (Katz, Ford, Moskowitz, Jackson, and Jaffe, 1963) in personal care areas are fairly easily modifiable through an intervention strategy utilizing reinforcement principles.

Basic principles of reinforcement involve strengthening new or appropriate behavior patterns while discouraging old or inappropriate patterns, through consistent application. For example, an aging person might refuse to eat at mealtime. It has been determined for this person that there is no physical problem that is preventing eating behavior, such as painful gums. Applying the principles of reinforcement, the paraprofessional might try complimenting the person every time eating occurred on its own, and might try ignoring the person when food was refused. It cannot be too strongly emphasized that reprimanding the person will not work. One reason for this is that a reprimand constitutes a form of attention, and attention given to a behavior will virtually insure its strengthening. In this example, then, attention given to not eating (via reprimand) would strengthen the very behavior that was targeted for elimination.

If the individual in the example above had been reinforced for eating and ignored for not eating by all staff in the treatment team, this would be a consistent application of the intervention strategy. However, if one day a new staff person reprimanded the individual for not eating, improvements that had been made on preceding days might be diminished. These principles will help paraprofessionals to be more effective change agents in a variety of situations with the aging. It is important to recognize that reinforcement is merely a tool, not to be used without first building a rapport with the client. That is, these principles are meant to be incorporated into normal daily therapeutic interventions in a natural, human style that communicates concern, warmth, and interest.

PSYCHOSOCIAL INTERVENTION THROUGH GROUP THERAPY

Psychosocial interventions encompassing eclectic treatment strategies are extremely effective with the aging when applied through group modalities. Some of these treatment modalities may be provided principally within institutions; other of these services may be provided within the community through a wide variety of federal, state, local, and privately funded programs. Just as with physical interventions, the paraprofessional never prescribes treatment programs but rather carries out designed programs under the supervision of a professional. A noncustodial approach applies to psychosocial as well as physical intervention, in that independent behaviors are encouraged with the goal of returning control of life events to the aging client, to the fullest possible extent. Psychosocial intervention, because it emphasizes the social interactive aspects of the client's problem, lends itself aptly and effectively to a group treatment strategy.

In some ways, the paraprofessional's group-leader role can be likened to the participant-observer role described in Chapter 6. In the group therapy setting, the participant observer acts as an active social facilitator for group interchanges. This reciprocal role allows participant observers to participate in the interaction while remaining aware that their mere presence qualitatively alters the outcome of the interaction. This interdependent criterion was first articulated by Lewin (1951) in his theory of group processes. The participant observer, as group leader, serves a different function than the traditional, noninvolved group leader, even though both may be engaged in the same pursuit (e.g., facilitating interaction among group members).

Important traits reported in the literature (Burnside, 1970) for the effective group leader with the aging are warmth, patience, flexibility, and perseverance, traits that should coincide with training goals for paraprofessionals. Whanger and Busse (1976) recommend that group leaders, preferably two to a group, take a positive and active role; the importance of a respectful, rather than casual, approach (preferably addressing the aging individual by surname) is emphasized. Added to the list of desirable group leader traits is, of course, genuine interest. Staff burnout, particularly where the group leaders take an active, verbal stance, is a serious deterrent to group progress, yet little is known to date about prevention. One way to avert burnout is for paraprofessional group leaders to keep themselves interested by introducing topics and activities that tap personal skills. For this reason, recreational group therapies are excellent treatment modalities that help prevent staff burnout while providing an activity framework for eclectic psychosocial intervention.

In some traditional therapies, the therapist and client do not make any physical contact; shaking hands might be the most affection expressed. The philosophical underpinnings of this non-touching premise involve issues of transference and maintenance of clear status delineations for alleged reasons of therapeutic effectiveness. There has lately come to the forefront another reason why some therapists resist touching their clients, involving misinterpretations of sexual advances by therapists toward clients, an issue that has more relevance for therapist and client of dissimilar gender. Touching has been advantageously used by Burnside (1973) as an adjunct to therapy with aging clients, serving the dual purpose of providing pleasurable, normal tactile feelings while communicating concern. This is extremely valued by the aging whose sensory losses may limit their range of experienced sensation, and who are often not given much attention other than that which goes with the custodial routine.

Group therapy is a realistic approach for the institutionalized aging because it allows for provision of treatment to a greatly expanded, otherwise ignored, number of clients (Wolff, 1967). Until very recently, the most popular, and often the only available, type of group therapy for the aging has been reality orientation.

This treatment provides reorientation through repetitions of basic information and discussions of graduated topics. This type of program, while quite effective in reorienting confused clients (Taulbee and Folsom, 1966; Birkett and Boltuch, 1973; Citrin and Dixon, 1975), is often perceived by aging clients as being below their level of competence. It is important that the specific problems of aging clients should be addressed in as insight-giving a manner as possible, as befits this elder population, despite mild or even moderate cognitive impairment. For example, sheltered workshops, initially introduced with the aging by Reingold and Wolk (1974), promote treatment designed to encourage meaningful task participation among aging clients. In one modified version of a sheltered workshop program (MacDonald and Settin, 1978), tasks were selected by group concensus, and where necessary, were adjusted to group members' physical capabilities. Sessions were held bi-weekly, each session lasting for approximately one hour and containing from six to ten group members. The components of the sessions were broken up into interdependent subparts in order to structurally encourage client interaction. The goals of this treatment were to promote social interaction, to increase the level of verbal behavior, to raise self-esteem through satisfaction in cooperative achievement, and to encourage independent behaviors.

The theory underlying these sheltered-workshop-type therapies is that the aging possess skills that may be lying dormant at this period of their lives and that can be reinitiated. Paraprofessionals can assist aging clients to rediscover the specific skills and talents, and make it possible for them to interact socially. It is unfortunately too often the case that these programs make only one or two tasks available, are short on materials and imagination, and more or less force the aging client into participating in something that is supposed to interest them. For example, groups for women almost always involve sewing, and those for men typically involve woodworking. The rehabilitative potential should reach far beyond to include athletic or calisthenic programs, art therapies, and so on.

The key to providing services for the aging is creativity. In this manner, any group therapy techniques that seem useful and appropriate for a client may be used in conjunction with one another. For example, music therapy is an effective yet greatly underutilized group intervention with the aging. It can provide socialization between various nationality/culture groups (including staff), physical exercise through use of rhythm instruments, foot tapping, hand clapping, personal satisfaction through regaining past musical skills, practice of verbal skills through singing, nostalgic recollection of old times (Shapiro, 1969; Shattin, Kotter, and Longmore, 1967). Similarly, art therapy can encourage expression of feelings in otherwise withdrawn nonverbal aging clients (Dewdney, 1973).

Milieu therapy, modeled after Jones' (1953) "therapeutic community", introduces a structured multi-level treatment program emphasizing self-management and community decision-making. Milieu therapy has been used with great success in a number of settings with the aging (Dubey, 1968; Gottesman, 1967; Goldstein, 1971; Birjani and Sclafani, 1973). Gottesman's program provided a "mixed-sex ward, a sheltered workshop doing paid industrial work, a ward store, frequent trips into the out-of-hospital community, and a program emphasizing patient responsibility for many aspects of their lives from self-care to partial operation of the workshop and the ward store." Ideally, the therapeutic milieu should continue outside the hospital as a transitional aftercare service. Despite the fact that Gottesman's program dates from 1967, little progress has been made in making these services available for the chronically institutionalized aging. This may be due to the fact that the utilization of milieu therapy requires highly integrated institutional support, making it a relatively complex innovation in traditional settings.

A promising direction for group therapy with institutionalized aging clients preparing for discharge is the predischarge therapy group. Adjustment problems following return to an alternative facility, a community placement, or family can be anticipated and explored. Paraprofessionals can function as important motivators in this process by providing supportive and informational counseling, helping the aging client to become aware of issues that may arise upon leaving the institution. Acting as case managers, paraprofessionals can assist by investigating needed support systems. Discussion groups typically deal with topics such as fear of independence, role-shift, financial management, loss of the familiar, and culture-shock resulting from long absence from a changed community.

Social-skills training, geared toward improving interpersonal relations, is indicated for the aging because they often have few social contacts, due to attrition of family and friends. The goal in social-skills training is to teach the client to be as effective as possible in social situations. This facilitates expression of social needs, enables true feelings and beliefs to be expressed in appropriate manner, and teaches assertiveness. By helping the aging to make active responses to situations and to be able to differentiate between aggressive and assertive behaviors, paraprofessionals can prepare clients to handle simulated situations that are difficult or anxiety-provoking for them. Social-skills training is effectively introduced in institutional settings when used in conjunction with some other treatment program, such as recreational therapy. However, paraprofessionals should be aware that the environment is not always supportive of appropriate assertive behavior, so that the theoretical merits of assertive behavior, for example, should be weighed against its possible negative consequences for the aging client.

In predischarge and social skills training groups, a useful strategy of intervention that can be employed by paraprofessionals is role play. Role play enables life situations to be simulated so that clients may see how their behavior appears to others, or so that clients may practice newly acquired behaviors. A specific situation is selected and the client is asked to act it out with one or more other group members, after which feedback is given by the group and moderated by the group leaders. Or, role reversal may be employed where two persons, for example the aging client and the paraprofessional, agree to exchange roles. The advantage to reverse-role playing is that it can not only reveal client behaviors and provide a means for modeling the more appropriate behavior for a client, but it can also show paraprofessionals how aging clients view them. Role play should be done in a nonevaluative, helpful manner and should always allow the client the opportunity to practice a behavior without fear of criticism. Perhaps the client typically uses an irritable tone of voice that alienates others, yet the client is unaware of this when it is brought up. By playing the staff, and replicating the tone of voice, the client can see how it sounds; by then playing the client and using a more pleasant tone of voice, the client can see that the "new" role is more effective. Role play used with videotape or audio-cassette feedback is an excellent therapy and training tool.

For the community aging undergoing a transitional or developmental crisis, such as death of a spouse (Morrice, 1976) or retirement (Caplan, 1964), crisis intervention clinics offer group and family therapy programs led by paraprofessionals. Through community clinics and area agencies on aging, crisis intervention is undergoing a rapid growth, and includes referral and information services as well as crisis counseling. Aging clients who need assistance in, for example, adapting to changes in role status or families of the aging concerned with health and welfare issues, are using these services readily. However, clinic utilization remains low, illustrating the cultural impediments (e.g., pride in solving one's own problems, fear of mental health problems, ignorance) that still exist for many aging persons in seeking out help. This underscores the need for outreach to access this needy and underserved aging population.

In summary, whether in an institutional or a community setting, supportive and goal-directed group therapy stressing development of competent coping strategies can be effectively carried out by trained paraprofessionals under the supervision of professionals. For example, one therapy goal might be directed toward remediation of age-associated losses, a prominent result of which can be depressed feelings and accompanying symptoms such as insomnia, loss of appetite, loss of interest in life, apathy or agitation, anger turned outward against others or inward toward self. Sharing of losses among group therapy members is an effective mode of treatment for such symptoms of depression; the feeling "I'm alone, no one understands my problems," can be experienced in the supportive group atmosphere, and possibly even resolved by process of mutual disclosure. Well-being is increased through an enhancement of interpersonal peer relations, and the group can serve an important function as a "surrogate family" for the aging. By utilizing a concrete, reality-based approach that allows the client to be expressive while at the same time obtaining feedback and practice in changing maladaptive behaviors, paraprofessionals can be effective in helping the aging to combat feelings of helplessness, dependency, inadequacy, and isolation.

Chapter 8

COGNITIVE-BEHAVIORAL
TECHNIQUES

COGNITIVE MODIFICATION

Cognitive impairments in aging clients, which are so mild as to be modifiable, are amenable to therapeutic intervention. That cognitive impairment (particularly in the area of intellectual performance) signals organic deterioration is common knowledge. Yet, emotional or psychological problems may also lead to decrements in intellectual performance (e.g., memory deficits). If performance anxiety can lower intelligence test scores for younger persons whose greater familiarity with testing situations should maximize performance, it stands to reason that aging persons who become anxious in evaluative situations, who are unfamiliar with testing, and generally more deliberate in their responses to novel material, should receive poorer test scores.

What of the aging with an affective illness, accompanied by impaired cognitive functioning? One proposed framework within which to view treatment of cognitive impairments is so-called cognitive modification (Meichenbaum and Cameron, 1973). Used successfully with young schizophrenic clients to improve intellectual performance, cognitive modification can provide a useful model for aging clients as well. According to these researchers, "Studies indicate that the schizophrenic's attentional and conceptual performance improve when the tasks involve stimulus refinement, such as reduced opportunities for distraction, or when the interpersonal conditions are perceived as nonthreatening, or when the schizophrenic receives immediate contingent feedback, or has a high drive level and is motivated. However, it appears unreasonable to expect a therapist to be able to engineer an environment, except within the limited conditions of a laboratory, where these conditions are continually met. Therefore it is necessary to consider an alternative treatment approach in which the schizophrenic patient is explicitly trained to provide his own attentional controls, to modify his own perceptions and motivation, to provide his own contingent feedback" (Meichenbaum and Cameron, 1973).

The stated problem with all therapies is that client behavior may be elicited only within the limited environment of the therapy session, and may not in fact generalize to situations outside the therapy surroundings. In a study investigating this problem of response generalization, Meichenbaum (1969) instructed an experimental group of schizophrenics to make a relevant, coherent speech response, called "healthy talk." The response generalization was observed to occur quite spontaneously; while showing improved performance on such conceptual tasks as word association and proverb interpretation, the schizophrenics used self-instructed cognitive assistance.

Meichenbaum and Cameron's (1973) "cognitive self-guidance" training technique was described as following five stages: (1) talking aloud by therapist while modeling task-relevant statements during task performance as client observes; (2) client performs task while therapist instructs aloud; (3) client performs task while providing own instructions aloud; (4) client performs task while whispering instructions; (5) client performs task covertly, giving instructions to self silently. The instructions were tailored to meet the clients' individual needs and included the necessary components of (a) question and answer to foster clear task instruction comprehension, (b) cognitive rehersal to focus on relevant task requirements and to prevent wandering of attention, (c) coping self-statements to handle frustration, and (d) self-reinforcement to maintain task perseverance.

Viewing verbal communication deficits as consequences of existing behavior-environment relationships in the institutional setting, Hoyer, Kafer, Simpson, and Hoyer (1974) successfully implemented operant procedures in the restatement of verbal behavior in aging, institutionalized schizophrenics, one of whom was characterized as not having talked for two years. One reason stated by the authors for utilizing behavior modification methods was that "these techniques may be implemented by paraprofessionals with effective training and supervision" (Hoyer et al., 1974). Similarly, reduced verbal behavior has been conceptualized as indicative of social isolation. A significant lessening in social isolation of residents of a nursing home measured by the rate of verbalization occurring around a dining-hall table was produced by prompting of speech followed by social reinforcement (e.g. smiling). "The simplicity of the procedure makes it suitable for geriatric facilities which are typically staffed by nonprofessional personnel" (MacDonald, 1978). This study also emphasizes the efficacy of employing behavioral as well as insight-oriented therapies with socially isolated, but otherwise normal, aging clients.

Treatment with the Cognitively Impaired Aging

In treatment with cognitively impaired aging clients, it is essential that a differential diagnosis be carried out by a professional, and that the relative degree of impairment be ascertained. The practical value of this is to counteract the assumption, held by many professionals (Wershow, 1977), that psycho-therapeutic management will not result in any significant reduction of symptoms. It is simply not the case that the only treatment for cognitively impaired aging clients is reality orientation alone, or custodial intervention designed to "maintain present level of functioning" or "prevent further deterioration."

Further, in any setting, there will exist misdiagnosed aging persons who will profit greatly from intervention. For example, Oberleder (1970) reports successful treatment and eventual discharge of twelve institutionalized aging clients (mean age 76 years), diagnosed as having chronic brain syndrome, with "crisis therapy" described as an "intensive treatment and practical action program." Treatment strategies with the cognitively impaired aging, because of accompanying changes in intellectual functioning, do indeed frequently require more concrete, briefer, non-insight-oriented therapies. The point is that clients should be given an adequate therapy trial before abandoning efforts in this direction. Paraprofessionals working with the cognitively impaired, or allegedly impaired, aging will probably be solely responsible for providing direct service intervention because few, if any psychotherapies are included in treatment plans for such clients.

The following case history and transcript illustrate the use of a verbal therapy with a severely impaired client.

> Mrs. R., a 65-year-old woman who worked as an executive secretary until the age of 62, underwent the death of her spouse, marriage of her daughter, and moving away of her son during the space of half a year. The onset of her illness at age 60 coincided with these events signaling important losses. She began drinking heavily alone, talked of suicide, had insomnia and intermittent memory loss, and presented a picture of severe depression for which she received various psychotherapies and medication. She lost her job because of gradually increasing dysfunctional work behavior, underwent screening for organic brain syndrome, and became a participant in an experimental university program for clients with senile dementia. Therapy having no result, she was moved to her daughter's home, where her gait became more unsteady and her memory worse over the course of the year. Finally, failing to recognize her daughter, yelling in the night and smearing feces, she was admitted to a psychiatric facility where she received several conflicting diagnoses, all reflecting some type of OBS. Suffering from peripheral neuropathy, she underwent an above-the-knee amputation rather

suddenly a year following admission. She was unable to cooperate with physical therapy staff, and subsequent attempts to fit her with a prosthesis were unsuccessful. She is now loudly talkative, brightly sociable, speech is echolalic and often word-salad. Her current diagnosis is Korsakov's psychosis, and she has been give up by staff: "Nothing can be done with her." She is confined for her own self-protection to a geriatric chair, where her incontinence naturally continues, and spends her entire day in a small room crowded with 20 other chairs. Seen twice weekly by psychologist for brief psychotherapy, she is quiet, attentive, and highly motivated to attend the sessions.

Transcript of a 15-minute session, conducted in a small private room off the day hall of the ward, occurring after six sessions:

T1: Hello, L.
C1: Hello. (smiles superficially)
T2: How are you feeling?
C2: Fine. (grimaces, looks down)
T3: Not so fine, maybe.
C3: Well, what do you you you there's a ting, ring a ting ting . . .
T4: It's hard to feel fine in a place like this.
C4: I'll say! (with feeling)
T5: Have you heard from S? (her daughter)
C5: (questioning look)
T6: She sent you a card for your birthday. I want to wish you a happy birthday too.
C6: My birthday? What a pretty blouse (reaches out to touch fabric)
T7: (smile) How old are you now?
C7: Sisisisisi . . . (other nonsensical speech)
T8: This is 1979, as I'm sure you know. That makes you 65 years old, but you look much younger.
C8: You're so nice (strokes sleeve of blouse)
T9: Thank you, L. Did you have a blouse like this when you worked?

C9: Many many baong bang bang bang . . . (loud)

T10: That was very loud.

C10: (silence)

T11: Have you been married, L?

C11: Oh my, yes. (drawn out)

T12: What was your husband's name?

C12: William. (tears come to eyes)

T13: T holds hand with C.

C13: Mother mother! (calling)

T14: You sound as if you feel abandoned, lonely. (Note: previously established ground rule—a nod can indicate response.)

C14: (no nod, stares hard directly at therapist)

T15: Remember, you don't have to speak, you can let me know how you feel by nodding like this. (demonstrates)

C15: Hmm. (looks away)

T16: You're not abandoned now.

C16: (nonsensical babbling)

T17: L, do you want to talk again sometime soon?

C17: You know I do.

T18: I like talking with you too. I'm going to be leaving now. See you in three days, on Thursday at two o'clock.

C18: Oh really? Good good good bye bye bye (other nonsensical speech)

Two major problems emerge in this type of exchange, the most troubling of which involves the need for therapist interpretation of most of this client's communications: the interpretation that tears in her eyes are in response to mention of her husband, that calling for mother is in response to being left alone, or that the client feels sad to be alone (not corroborated by client). Does lack of confirmation in response to this therapist mean that no comprehension of the directions to nod has occurred? Was the client really sad, or is this countertransference on the part of the therapist?

The other problem involves the directive nature of therapist's questions, and the effect this has on the client: bringing in old material in the form of a question about her husband, since this exchange has taken place before. Yet, the client responds similarly in each session to mention of her husband, which can be taken as some confirmation that this response is indicative of genuine comprehension of the question. Might this material not be too stressful for the client, in the absence of more intensive exploration available to a more verbal client? To monitor the client's behavior for signs of stress, a paraprofessional therapy aide has been asked to spend 15 minutes a day at the same time sessions normally occur. This has the advantage of providing a second object for attention (the first being the therapist) and of providing companionship therapy.

In this type of therapy, the therapist must hold certain beliefs about the client: (a) that client is capable of understanding communications, (b) that client is able to give appropriate nonverbal responses, even if the verbal responses are inappropriate, (c) that client enjoys the encounter with the therapist, and (d) that client benefits from expressing emotion. The goals of the early sessions with this client were to establish rapport, to give the client "permission" to say or do anything she likes with the understanding that therapist will come back, and to treat client's nonsensical, echolalic speech as real communications having a beginning and end, enabling her to finish without interruption and to respond to the nonverbally expressed emotion as if she had expressed it verbally.

It was important in designing the treatment strategy for Mrs. R. to provide immediate contingent feedback toward modification of the inappropriate behavior she exhibited (e.g., echolalic, nonsensical speech). It was found that touching was a strong reinforcer for this client, a behavior she emitted frequently by herself. By ignoring the inappropriate speech while focusing on the underlying feeling of the speech rather than the overt "sick talk" content, and by giving feedback in the form of touching (defined as enabling the client to touch the therapist's arm and hand, or holding her hand), the frequency of "sick talk" gradually decreased in the therapy setting. It should be noted, however, that no noticeable change in behavior occurred in the day hall. Again, the problem of response generalization points up the bond between environment and behavior. In order to promote generalization, a paraprofessional therapy aide was instructed to use touching as social reinforcement in the day hall for appropriate verbal communication.

This client was later able to enter into a group therapy treatment program, with her paraprofessional therapy aide as group leader, without exhibiting disruptively loud verbal behaviors. While her degree of cognitive impairment remained constant, her social behavior was more adaptive (e.g. elicited positive responses from staff and group members), and her daughter reinitiated occasional visits. In discussing techniques used with confused aging patients, Yalom and Terrazas (1968) conclude that group therapy "has much to offer the psychotic elderly patient. By setting realistic goals, by increasing patient interaction, by focusing on patient strengths and similarities, and by building group cohesiveness, the therapist can demonstrate that pessimism about group therapy with this population is unwarranted."

The operant view of treatment has been suggested by Hoyer, Mishara, and Riebel (1975) as a useful conceptual model for treating many problem behaviors of the aging institutionalized client: "Regardless of whether reinforcement principles are employed, the emphasis placed on the measurement of observable behavior, and on the individualization of treatment (in terms of what is effective for changing that individual's behavior) has implications for most if not all therapeutic attempts with elderly persons" (Hoyer, Mishara, and Riebel, 1975). Like any therapeutic technique, behavior modification is only effective and ethical when used skillfully and appropriately, with discretion and sensitivity to the client's needs. Viewed within its proper perspective, that of its value to the client, it can be of particular usefulness to the aging.

For example, Mishara, Robertson, and Kastenbaum(1973) observed that staff were giving more attention to self-injurious behavior of the aging than to nondestructive behaviors. In other words, reinforcement was being given for undesirable behaviors, in an attempt by staff to stop them, but clearly of negative outcome for the client. By training staff to ignore negative attention-seeking behaviors, and to reinforce positive behaviors, the incidence of self-injurious behavior decreased. Contingency management, or "operant" techniques, were also used by Geiger and Johnson (1974) who succeeded in improving eating behavior in aging clients who had previously eaten less than 50 percent of their meals. Reinforcers, which were desired things selected by the clients themselves, were administered contingent upon correct eating. It is suggested that paraprofessional staff be trained in effective positive management procedures, such that "more productive behaviors for elderly persons might be achieved, and misuse of this or other management techniques can be discouraged" (Geiger and Johnson, 1974).

A behavioral approach with the aging is practical if viewed from no other perspective than promoting the likelihood that staff will interact more often in a change-worthy way with the aging. The persistent stereotype of the aging, that they are too old to change, has infiltrated the institution where staff maintain attitudes that merely reflect the current, negative, societal view. It is true that the aging suffer from more physical disability than other-aged populations, realistically requiring more custodial treatment that can preclude provision of much-needed treatment for psychological or emotional problems. However, it is more the case that staff give up on the aging client, because "they are just going to die anyhow," or "they are only senile" (to borrow a chapter heading from Robert Butler's (1975) impassioned plea for equitable treatment of the aging: "Why Survive: Being Old in America"). Such negative feelings about the aging virtually ensure their lack of treatment, which in turn, ensures their decline.

By graphically illustrating that staff can intervene successfully with problem behaviors (such as incontinence, incorrect eating, self-injurious behavior, social isolation), behavioral procedures show that the aging under their care can change, and what is more, that staff themselves help them to do so. There is no "professional mystique" about implementation of behavioral procedures; in fact, behavioral researchers have gone out of their way to suggest that a principal advantage of the procedure is that paraprofessionals can be "behavioral engineers" of the treatment team. Thus, the role of the paraprofessional working with the aging has been expanded by behavioral technology to include the tasks of: (1) providing reinforcement using available stimuli (e.g. social reinforcement) in the therapy setting to promote response generalization across environments; (2) monitoring client behavior for critical change; (3) measuring client responses to determine degree of change induced by the treatment.

A COGNITIVE PROSTHESIS FOR THE AGING

Even though the aging individual may carry an organic diagnosis, there exists the possibility that a mixed diagnosis or an incorrect diagnosis has unwittingly condemned the client to an inappropriate treatment modality. Too often, the truth is that professionals base their intervention strategies upon the assigned diagnosis rather than the observed behavior. It may be that a cognitively oriented approach would have been effective with a client, but was not tried because of a presumed inability to process information adequately. It is here proposed that maladaptive coping strategies account for much of the "problem behavior" exhibited by the aging, both within and without institutions, and that training the aging in coping strategies need not require total cognitive integrity.

Meichenbaum (1974) has proposed a cognitive prosthesis for the aging, which goes far in addressing this need for practical application of coping strategies. The cognitive prosthesis involves an adaptation of the "cognitive self-guidance training technique" in combination with a modified systematic desensitization procedure, with the goal of teaching the aging client specific coping strategies. Such strategies are, for example, taking slow deep breaths, or giving self-instructions for feedback.

One value of the cognitive prosthesis lies in its having solved the problem of response generalization, wherein the client's skills acquired within the therapy setting fail to be maintained in their "normal" environment (e.g., outside the therapy room). By providing self-reinforcement, the client is not dependent upon others for the maintenance of the new behavior or skill. Another value lies in the training of self-administered cues that eventually come to induce an internal climate for producing adaptive behaviors. A third value is that the strategy treats thoughts as well as actions. For those persons who achieve insight into the effect of, for example, maladaptive thoughts upon their actions, so much the better; for those who do not achieve insight, thoughts can be dealt with as concrete entities that can be modified. A fourth value is the greatly positive view the cognitive prosthesis holds of virtually every aging client's capabilities. That it can be introduced in stages according to the specific needs of that client, by trained paraprofessionals, in any setting, makes it one of the single most impressive treatment strategies yet seen for the aging.

Chapter 9

ENVIRONMENTAL DESIGN

AN HOLISTIC CONCEPT

Environmental design is a concept referring to the planning of new systems to meet individual needs (Barker, 1968). It is a broad definition taking into account the individual's total "life space" in conjunction with architectural, economic, political, and social factors. By this definition, anything that affects the individual is environmental, and anything that is changed in the environment by intention is environmental design. Because environmental design means any planned change in the environment, therapeutic intervention might also be considered part of designed environments, where, for example, group interventions bring aging persons together to practice new skills.

Interrelating aspects of environment are: (1) the individual environment, which includes physical capabilities; (2) the social environment, which includes family, friends, acquaintances, health paraprofessionals (participant observers); (3) the physical environment, which includes external factors (such as the design of housing) and internal factors (such as interior design). Applying

108

this to the specific case of an aging person suffering from visual impairment or restricted mobility, an environmental design solution would be: (1) individual environment: eyeglasses, walker; (2) social environment: others describe details that aging person cannot see, participation in exercise groups; (3) physical environment: appliances with Braille controls, ramps instead of steps. Such environmental-design solutions may seem self-evident, yet many of these prophylactic and rehabilitative steps are not available for the community aging, and are often not even implemented within institutions.

An explanation for the lack of acceptance of the notion of environmental design within institutions may be found in an examination of the organizational structure and economic motivation of the total institution. The structure of the total institution places a low priority on intervention, particularly for low-status individuals such as the aging. Intervention aimed at shortening the individual's stay conceivably threatens the future of the facility. Another explanation for nonimplementation of environmental design is the misunderstanding that it merely encompasses the physical properties of a setting. Further, the concept of illness as residing with the individual is still common despite decades of research focusing on person/environment interactions as determinants of behavior.

The primary task of the environmental designer is to understand the environment and to create new environmental systems to meet the individual's needs (Sanoff and Cohen, 1969). In this sense, paraprofessionals are environmental designers, observing, understanding, creating environments for the aging. "Person condition interactions are never static, but environmental stabilities can be identified which help to account for continuities in behavior and permit useful precisions" (Mischel, 1973).

INDIVIDUAL ENVIRONMENTS

Cautela's (1972) contention that "such behaviors as 'lack of enthusiasm' or 'aimless talking, walking and moving' are primarily due to lack of adequate stimulus variability and reinforcement of activity" where "proper manipulation of environmental stimuli can often reduce inactive behavior" expresses the fundamental notion in environmental design of the causative role played by the environment in sensory deprivation. Within institutions, continued exposure to poor lighting, lack of color, dimensionless shape, and flat texture can lead to depression. Reminiscing may be explained in part by the need to supply stimulation in terms of fantasies when stimulation is not supplied from outside either because of sensory deficits or designer deficits, or both.

Protheses for reducing sensory deficits are part of the aging person's individual micro-environmental design. For example, hearing aids and glasses, artificial limbs, canes, walkers, wheelchairs, and orthopedic shoes require diagnosis of a sensory deficit before the next step of intervention can be taken. Schwartz (1975) lists the category of furniture in illustrating the "penalizing" environment confronting the aging, such as heavy doors, inaccessible storage space, and so on. Prosthetic compensation for deficits enhances individual effectiveness, supports competence, and maintains self-esteem (Lindsley, 1964). For the aging, who have a higher incidence of both sensory and social deprivation than any other age group, failure to remediate problems in the sensory realm will herald extreme withdrawal and possibly precipitate serious emotional disturbances.

SOCIAL ENVIRONMENTS

Useful in the conceptualization of social withdrawal is the notion of social velocity (Calhoun, 1963), relating to identifying properties in the environment that enhance or detract from the probability that social interaction will occur. As early as 1950, social psychologists became interested in the impact of environment, specifically residential design, on social systems. Results of their investigations showed that local friendship-network development was enhanced by the proximity of apartments. Later studies indicated that local social networks suffer from architectural rather than spatial design characteristics such as long corridors and high-rise apartments (Davis and Baum, 1975). An interaction between architectural and interior design and the social environment characterized by low social velocity describes the typical situation for the aging both within and without institutions. The aging have relatively few opportunities for social interaction; when interaction occurs it may do so in spite of the environment. For example, a social interaction group for aging inpatients is held in a narrow rectangular room so that participants sit in rows rather than in the more communication-facilitating circle.

Environmental intervention has been so successful with the aging in promoting social interaction (Kastenbaum, 1968) because it is goal-directed and based upon observable behaviors. This enables paraprofessionals to work with concrete guidelines toward attainable goals. Once the goal is identified, it can be readily adapted into different treatment strategies. For example, the specific treatment goal of increased social interaction might be realized by designing environments that reinforce or facilitate interpersonal interactions in quantifiable amounts. Integration of sex-segregated wards (Silverstone and Winter, 1975), serving wine (Mishara and Kastenbaum, 1974), beer (Berker and Cesar, 1973; Chien, 1971) or the introduction of any novel stimulus have all significantly increased rates of social interaction.

If such interventions enhance the behavioral repertoire so easily, it may seem puzzling to consider why they are not routine parts of every institutional environment. First of all, these interventions may be simple in theory, but they are not in fact simple to implement. Any change in routine necessitating staff involvement will be extremely difficult to effect unless it is recognized, from the administrator on down, as being a requirement. When analysed in terms of power relationships, it can be seen that it would be preferable even in merely moving a chair from one location to another, that the change be generated by staff. Further, despite the fact that wine, for example, has been used successfully before, its introduction may violate the letter (if not the spirit) of the law. These factors mitigate against innovation, and go far in explaining why environmental-design notions may require careful introductory ground work before being accepted.

Physical Environments

Physical design of the environment is important for the aging not only for aesthetic or prophylactic reasons, but for reasons of safety as well. For example, the aging person who has difficulty walking is more likely to slip and fall if halls are narrow and poorly lit, and floors are slick and waxed (MacDonald and Butler, 1973). Wheelchair-confined persons are totally unable to get out without ramps. An environmental-design solution would be to provide the person with rubber-soled shoes, to light hallways adequately, and to cover waxed floors with runners. This would result in increased mobility, social activity (e.g., visiting a neighbor), and generally better physical and psychological health.

Sommer and Ross (1958) were among the first environmental designers to investigate the effects on morale of changing the physical environment. By rearranging lobby furniture so that chairs faced one another, and by using round instead of rectangular tables, morale (defined as frequency of conversation between residents) was significantly increased. McClannahan and Risley (1975) placed a shopping area in a nursing-home lobby, increasing residents' use of this space and implying that residents thus increased their level of physical activity. However, these outcomes of merely rearranging space may be short-lived effects, and physical spatial change alone may represent an insufficient condition for change in resident behavior. In other words, individuals need to not only be brought together in the appropriate physical setting but must also have prompting or reinforcement of the desired behavior (Snyder, 1973) in order to produce long term changes in behavior.

In reviewing these studies, caution should be exercised in discarding what might at first seem to be negative or nonsignificant results of some environmental designs. For example, Lawton, Liebowitz, and Charon (1970) implemented an extensive, ward-wide remodeling program, incorporating a variety of sound principles of environmental design. Residents responded within the environmental design area by being less physically active and less socially responsive; upon closer examination of the data, residents were shown to have improved on these two dimensions outside of the environmental design area. This interesting finding was interpreted in a positive light as demonstrataing increased perception of control over the environment that ensued from the remodeling program.

Housing for the aging has received a great deal of deserved attention in the past decade. Lipman and Slater (1977) outline architectural blueprints for housing that are models of thoughtful individual, social and physical design for the aging (for example, ramps replace stairs). Further, architects support the idea that "what a physical setting will do to behavior of the people using that space is not simply a result of the number of square feet available to each person, the floor plan, or the color of the wall" (Ostrander, 1973). Thus, while the architectural design is important, the neighborhood and site location is no less so. It would of course be desirable for the aging to remain in their old familiar neighborhoods. However, places change over time, once-supportive neighborhoods deteriorate, friends and family relocate or die, to the point where there is no longer a sense of community. Again, perceived control over one's housing, neighborhood, and personal environment is an important determinant of satisfaction.

A major social problem having great impact on neighborhood relocation, fear of crime, is ranked by the aging at the top of the list, even above health (Harris, 1975; Toseland and Rasch, 1978), despite the fact that the aging are actually the least likely group to be victimized (Cook, Skogan, Cook and Antunes, 1978). Ironically, a recent study reveals that community housing is actually safer (e.g., measured by a lower reported crime rate) than age-segregated housing (Kahana, Liang, Felton, Fairchild, and Harel, 1977). The aging tend to move more often as a result of ill health,

loss of job, or loss of spouse (Steinfeld, 1977) than in response to
fear of crime. When relocation occurs, the important issue for the
aging in one study was not accessibility or cost of services, but
rather neighborhood characteristics (Lawton, Brody, and Turner-
Massey, 1976).

The aging in rural settings suffer similar breakdowns in health
and social networks necessitating relocation, including one critical
problem not confronted by the urban aging: mobility. Transportation is becoming an increasing problem, with rising cost of insur-
ance, fuel, and upkeep for private vehicles. The majority use
public transportation, which could not be utilized by fully 40% of
urban aging in one study (Stirner, 1978) who were handicapped
and 6% who were nonambulatory, and the remaining 54% might
not be able to negotiate poor design features such as high bus steps.
Socialization opportunities may be sharply curtailed without a car
or public transportation and aging persons may have to increasingly depend on others to take them shopping and even to visit a
friend. Lack of mobility is a serious deterrent to health, since
psycho-social, medical, and dental services cannot then be utilized
with any regularity. Stirner (1978) also found that 30% need
additional transportation, the majority of these indicating the
reason as visit to clinic or doctor.

Control and predictability are variables identified as accounting for a significant amount of variability in the physical and
psychological status of the aging (Schultz, 1975; Stone and Kranz,
1976). Perceived control over the impinging environment can lead
to the aging person's initiation of coping behaviors. "Learned
helplessness" is a passive psychological problem based upon dependency and powerlessness. Restricting the individual's freedom
of choice directs the "environmental press" toward learned helplessness and other negative expressions of stress (Birren and Renner, 1976; Calhoun, 1962; Maier and Seligman, 1976). Even the
community aging are deprived of at least one or more of these
factors necessary for dignity: sensory stimulation, physical activity, social interaction, privacy, meaningful activity, social status—in other words, control over their environment.

It is not possible for environmental design intervention to redress deprivation arising from objective realities of aging, such as fear of crime or lack of mobility, and status once lost is hardly recoverable. However, implementation of environmental design concepts can prevent further deprivation. Environmental design paraprofessionals could be trained to function in community settings (such as universities, nutrition sites, congregate housing sites) that involve systematic planning of total environments toward participant observation of relations between environmental variables and behavior change.

Chapter 10

ALTERNATIVES TO INSTITUTIONALIZATION

DEINSTITUTIONALIZATION

The national policy termed "deinstitutionalization" of transferring residents, particularly aging residents, from mental institutions into the community, was heralded by social planners as a necessary theoretical step toward community health. However, in practice, the process was "carried out precipitously, hazardously, and inhumanly" (Donahue, 1977). At the height of this process in the early 1970's, the deinstitutionalized aging were commonly transferred to nursing or adult homes that were often more restrictive settings than the mental institution from which they came (Markson, Levitz, and Gognalons-Caillard, 1973; Brill, 1979). Adult homes, with substandard housing or inadequate nutritional programs, were the most frequent recipients for "dumping"; the community was entirely unprepared for the arrival of these deinstitutionalized, but otherwise unchanged, residents (Brill, 1979). This population thus ended up back in the mental institution in considerably worse shape than prior to discharge, except for those who died as a result of premature relocation.

On the other hand, the adverse impact on the aging of prolonged institutionalization should not be ignored. MacDonald (1973) has outlined multiple contributors to the deleterious effects of prolonged nursing home residence. Among these, the "sick role" ascribed to the aging as a result of their institutionalization is particularly salient. While it is obviously important not to lodge the aging inappropriately in institutions when they could receive treatment in a community setting, "The absence of supportive services and alternative living arrangements has created an erosion in the middle level of care" (Brill, 1979) that makes remediation of this problem impossibly difficult. State mental institutions thus continue to provide a needed setting for indigent aging persons who have no visible means of support or whose benefits are insufficient to maintain them in the community.

Given this quandary, it would be naive not to endorse the legitimate need for long-term-care institutions. But more importantly, there will always be a percentage of the aging population who require total institutionalization by reason of the severity of their disabilities. It is becoming increasingly clear that advocates for the elimination of long-term-care are taking a facile approach to a complex problem. It is too easy to criticize long-term-care systems or, for that matter, to criticize society at large. Many of these criticisms are valid; however, they are quickly tempered by visits to deteriorated adult homes, custodial care nursing homes, or single-room-occupancy hotels used unsuccessfully as urban dumping sites.

The aging in institutions are more realistic than many social planners about their alternatives. An actual case in point was a 73-year-old recovering alcoholic, psychiatric resident for the past 24 years, in good physical and psychological health, who was interviewed by a social worker. Asked whether he would like to be discharged he replied, "I'd have to be crazy to want to stay in this dump, and I'd be a damn fool to leave. I get a room, three meals a day, and nobody bothers me." This indigent aging man has been twice refused for family care because of his history of alcoholism; he has also been refused for discharge to a nursing facility as a transitional step because he carries a psychiatric rather than physical diagnosis. Merely discharging people into the community is just not a viable response to what has become an increasingly serious social problem complicated by lack of housing, inflation, and other objective socio-environmental conditions existing in the community.

Preparatory efforts to deinstitutionalize residents from long-term-care facilities have focused upon the concept of transitional service. The transitional component involved special retraining and rehabilitation of the aging for preparation for community discharge. This often meant rigorous screening procedures prior to entering rehabilitation programs, long stays in sheltered workshops while continuing institutional living, and finally movement out into the community on a day-pass basis to further continue sheltered workshops and other rehabilitative pursuits. For most persons enrolled in predischarge programs within long-term-care facilities this was as far as the discharge process could lead. The logical next step of discharge, while difficult enough to effect with younger persons, is practically impossible with the aging. This is not necessarily because the aging have spent too many years housed in institutions or because they have irrevocably lost adaptive skills as a result of neglect. It is perhaps because of community resistance against the deinstitutionalized (Brill, 1979), yet other deinstitutionalized groups such as the mentally retarded have been able (albeit with difficulty) to overcome community prejudice. The most serious problem is that these aging have no source of income other than government subsidy, have lost their social-support systems, and simply have no place to live.

RESIDENTIAL ALTERNATIVES

In response to this need, family residences (foster care) and group homes have emerged as a viable alternative. These residences offer a normalizing, less restrictive rehabilitative alternative to institutionalization. In one such family home in New York State, no more than three aging persons, who must be ambulatory, not dangerous to self or others, free from alcohol or substance dependency, not in need of skilled nursing, and voluntary, live full-time with a host family selected by the family residencial agency. They can originate from psychiatric facilities (deinstitutionalized aging persons) or the community (aging with a history of mental or emotional disability). The family members enter into a contractual agreement where support, training, and formal clinical evaluation are the responsibility of the residencial agency's clinical staff. In effect, the members of the host family, an already existing resource, are paraprofessionals. Family or group homes, in addition to providing the aging with a needed alternative to total institutionalization, can also provide meaningful, gainful employment for established, community-dwelling aging homeowners. Kirby, Polak, and Deever (1975) found greater improvement in "mentally ill" clients assigned randomly to a family home compared with a psychiatric institution; chief reasons cited were the de-objectification of the individual and the structural integration of client with "helper."

The concept of residential homes for the aging is viable in a rural setting, but no parallel residential alternative has been proposed for urban settings. For example, a single-room-occupancy (SRO) hotel in a city provided a model for developing comprehensive treatment and rehabilitation programs for aging welfare residents and deinstitutionalized psychiatric patients (Plutchik, McCarthy, Hall, and Silverberg, 1973). Services provided were medical, psychiatric, recreational, and social, aimed at providing improved quality of life and establishing a sense of community and personal autonomy among residents. Two important features of the program were the utilization of paraprofessionals as intervention agents and advocates, and the implementation of a job core providing salaries for a small number of residents at jobs within the hotel. A full-time alcoholism counselor, a 24-hour crisis intervention counseling service, and a floor counselor were other important features of the program.

Unfortunately, this project, like most others of its genre, suffered from funding cutbacks and from changes in welfare policies, which no longer make it possible for the aging to be discharged under such programs with adequate support. It is felt that attempts at coordinated services such as the "hotel model" go far in providing multi-modal residential services so needed by the aging following discharge. And, it would enable the aging from urban areas to be discharged back into a familiar community, which would facilitate adjustment.

PREVENTION

The other side of the coin from deinstitutionalization is prevention: prevention of institutionalization. Prevention can be conceptualized as a viable model for maintaining the independence of "high risk" aging before they become so debilitated due to lack of support services in the community that they require total institutionalization. Prevention with the aging can be conceptualized as either primary or secondary, primary entailing prevention of the inception of physical or psychological problems through programs of education and immunization, and secondary prevention entailing early detection of illness and control of its progress through treatment. It is this secondary-prevention framework that has proved a most effective concept in implementing community services for the aging designed to prevent the need for total institutionalization.

Neighborhood service centers, outgrowths of community mental-health programs, are particularly desirable because they reflect the specific needs of the indigent aging populations, which vary from community to community. Neighborhood service centers focus on the central role played by the small group in community life, and introduce external leadership around whom indigenous paraprofessional leaders can be rallied as service providers. Importantly, the aging are not treated within this intervention strategy as "ill" or "frail" but rather as normal members of society with a particular set of social problems attendant upon aging. Paraprofessionals can often be more effective than professionals because they function as a "bridge between a low income population and the middle class professional" (Peck, Kaplan, and Roman, 1966) and because being from the community they have access to knowledge about nontraditional local support modalities that professionals might not be aware of.

Based on a storefront walk-in concept, the neighborhood center is advertised to community residents as a place to come in time of crisis, for sources of information about psychological, physical, and social problems, for guidance in dealing with red tape (for example, in making Medicare/Medicaid application). The goal is to provide easy access support, and referral for treatment where necessary, to enable continued community residence for the aging. An example of one successful storefront center for the aging (Santore and Diamond, 1974), which was staffed by aging paraprofessionals, involved social-action programs (one of which brought about the relocation of inaccessible food-stamp centers). The storefront concept is important for the reason that (a) it requires little funding and can rely heavily upon local resources of paraprofessional volunteers while being run by trained health paraprofessionals, and (b) because it can be physically located adjacent to oft-used centers within the community to maximize visibility and facilitate utilization by the aging.

The extension of the community mental-health center has been the multi-service center. Such centralized organizations have ambitious goals, are extremely expensive to set up and run, and are then underutilized. They also tend to be superimposed upon the community more or less regardless of the aging population's requirements within this community. Multi-service center objectives (Gurian and Scherl, 1972) are typically to: (a) provide comprehensive mental-health services directly and indirectly through consultation; (b) develop and implement training programs for persons involved with the aging; (c) create a home base for organization and action by the aging themselves, (d) implement program evaluation and need-assessment surveys. What generally happens with such centers is that they have the capacity for provision of excellent direct health intervention, assessment, and training programs; however, the indirect service and advocacy portions suffer since direct service needs invariably expand too rapidly for the budget.

It is unfortunate that community multi-service centers in America do not follow the pattern established in England, Denmark, and the Netherlands where paraprofessionals from indigent target communities serve their own target populations with efficiency and economy. One such model British community center (Robinson, 1969) provides an excellent outreach screening program in addition to above-mentioned functions. Annual home visits are made to every aging person in the catchment area for prevention and remediation followed by referrals where necessary. In addition, supportive services are thorough and creative, combining home nursing, volunteer helpers, speech and occupational therapy, transportation aides, meals on wheels, visiting libraries, and so on.

Outreach is beginning to gain popularity in the United States, although it will undoubtedly suffer from the same problems encountered by other prevention programs: lack of political support, lack of funding, and poor organization. Outreach has gained popularity partially in response to the widespread failure of practically all other alternatives to institutionalization, and the need to service adequate numbers of community aging. The problem of underutilization of services by the aging target population is extremely serious, particularly for the rural aging. For example, many aging have no transportation, which should lead policy planners toward improving the location of preventive services and increasing public awareness of the existence of such services (Meeker, 1976).

The concept of the outreach worker is familiar to persons who work with paraprofessionals in civic, religious, and social-welfare organizations, yet it has until recently been an alien concept in the allied health professions. Outreach fills the multiple function of (1) providing checkup services for that hidden majority of community aging who are marginally functional and at high risk for physical and psychological problems that will lead to disability if untreated.

The first step is to identify the existence of such individuals, the second is to find out what they need and want in the way of assistance, and the third is to provide it. This strategy is at the core of every community health program yet few programs have been able to surmount the administrative staffing difficulties involved in running a large outreach organization. As a result, outreach programs are typically staffed by volunteers and paraprofessionals, or are run by nonprofit civic associations.

Many aging persons cannot function independently in their homes because they have not been trained in the use of assistive devices, techniques of self-care, and self-medication. According to Hudson (1974), a program of routine (e.g. once per month) home visits by paraprofessionals trained by professional staff in maximizing existing potential for independent living could have prevented a number of disabling accidents. Paraprofessionals could perform a variety of case management functions, including ongoing social contact, scheduling and arranging of transportation, in-house chore and resident services, escort for referral to other supportive services, and many others.

Examples of such supportive programs for the community aging are: home repairs, dial-a-ride, senior companions, shopping assistance, tutorial services, merchandise and drug delivery, and visiting home health services. Home health services have existed for many years under the auspices of such agencies as the Visiting Nurse Service. One such program (Berg, Atlas, and Zeiger, 1974) trained paraprofessionals to travel to the home to provide maintenance services such as shopping, cleaning, and food preparation. The paraprofessionals involved could respond to the needs of their service population in a situation where the professional could not. An important psychosocial treatment function served by the home-visiting paraprofessional is provision of reality-testing opportunities and reduction of isolation through consistent contact for the aging homebound with the outside world.

Recognizing that lack of meaningful activity is one of the greatest problems confronting the aging today, agencies are being formed by the aging for the aging. RSVP (Retired Senior Volunteer Program) provides services on a regular basis to community agencies and arranges for placement, training, and transportation to volunteer assignments. The Gray Panthers, an organization of both young and old dedicated to combating ageism, has its greatest strength in provocation of social change. A program of foster grandparents provides the aging with the oportunity to serve in hospitals and other institutions in return for a stipend, transportation allowance, annual physical examination, and daily free meals. These programs are an exciting combination of an important human resource, the aging paraprofessional, and a needed service for the aging.

More home-service providers exist in rural areas, because outreach programs were first developed for use in inaccessible geographic regions (e.g., Appalachia, the Dust Bowl region of the Midwest). What is too often forgotten is that urban environments can be as inaccessible and alienating as hills or deserts. The numbers of neglected aging living in crowded apartment buildings in cities or run-down garden apartments in suburbs have not been accurately determined. Informal sources report the overwhelming crisis conditions under which such aging persons live, with too little food and clothing, no telephone, no support networks. Therefore, contrary to the popular notion that the family is quick to shift its ailing aging to institutions, many impaired aging remain at home, cared for by their families in "one-bed hospitals" (Bell, 1973).

For such infirm aging, (Bell, 1975) reports a community service utilizing a converted school bus as a mobile medical screening service. Approximately 3,000 persons were serviced during the first half year of operation and 13% of these were referred for further treatment. Systematic screening and evaluation of the aging person's current functional status will expedite identification of problem areas in the realm of physical, psychological, and nursing needs, communication skills, family relationships, and physical environment. A second type of mobile geriatric team might originate within state departments of mental health, or private hospitals, to provide screening, intervention, liaison, and resource functions for the aging within that hospital's catchment area. A team would consist of interchangeable professionals (e.g. psychologist, community mental-health nurse, physician, social worker), and paraprofessionals. The first function, screening, would involve a careful determination of the nature of the medical, psychological, and social problems that have brought that particular aging person to the team's attention.

A thorough functional assessment of a young person is performed as a matter of course, but aging persons are too often passed over perfunctorily in examination. This is particularly important in light of the fact that the aging, if only by way of their having lived a greater number of years and been ill or infirm more often, will probably have a greater number of problems to evaluate. Time and other environmental constraints imposed upon the clinical team entering a community setting to perform the evaluation dictate that a standardized format be followed. The evaluation should consist of information including (1) health status—medical history, diet, medication regime, appraisal of current abilities (especially ADL), physical examination including pulse, blood pressure, temperature, mobility, referral for appropriate laboratory testing, nursing-care-needs appraisal; (2) mental status—history, reported and observed behavior, affective state, intellectual function (memory, concentration), communication, orientation, psychological judgment and insight, cognitive impairment, ability to comprehend and use language, sensory acuity, hand/eye coordination, ability to abstract and categorize information; (3) social environment—capability and willingness of family and/or friends to help, insight of family into problems, level of social interaction; (4) physical environment—adequacy of housing, proximity to services, safety, general organization of environment to meet needs, transportation, noise, pollution; (5) quality of life.

On the basis of this assessment, a decision would then be reached about the kind of care, if any, needed by the client and where that care could be provided in the least restrictive environment. Following these evaluations, a coordinated team plan for future management would be worked out with the aging person, or those who are responsible for the aging person, and with the family. The most practical plan may not always be the ideal plan. For example, the aging person may live next door to the hospital and the most practical plan might then be viewed as acute care via institutionalization, even when the aging individual could remain in the community and utilize supportive community services.

The individual would be assessed on-site so that family members are included in the decision, and so that behavioral assessment can be made of the individual within the environmental context of the community. The team would also function as a referral source and would be familiar with the facilities and services available for the aging in their community. Follow-up procedures would also be established, including re-examination date, following the practice of sending a reminder notice prior to the appointment. The team's role would not be confined to consultation in individual cases but would also involve consultation to staff of other institutions (such as nursing homes) and the organization of educational programs for the community it serves.

The obvious advantage of an institution-based mobile geriatric team is that it would allow for continuity of care and reciprocity among service delivery agencies. For example, a nursing home may call in the team to screen a resident who evidences indications of mental disability. Upon screening, the team may recommend brief psychiatric hospitalization, which under this program would last for six weeks before re-evaluation toward discharge would take place. Ideally, the same personnel who staff the screening team would also staff the admissions unit in the state hospital. Hospital staff would be trained in aging and preventive community health-service concepts. Discharge planning would be supervised by a screening team with prior knowledge, for example, that a particular environment precipitated deterioration, thereby reducing the likelihood of return through that particular "revolving door." Or the screening team may be called in by the family of an aging person and upon assessment and discussion with the family, the aging person may not require institutionalization. Appropriate referral to community-based supportive services may instead be made. The screening team would retain this person's record, enabling a routine follow-up visit to take place.

An alternate mode of outreach suggested by Kushler and Davidson (1978) and successfully employed by Cohen (1974) involves linking outreach with information and referral services. One such service was "CRISIS" (Counseling, Referral & Information Service for Seniors), an experimental hotline for the aging (Settin and Julius, 1977). The service originated as a small volunteer project staffed and run exclusively by undergraduate-student paraprofessionals to provide services to needy and high-risk community aging. Phase I of the project involved (a) development of a ten-week, 20-hour training program oriented toward interviewing techniques emphasizing discrimination and attending, after Carkhuff's (1969) well-known training paradigm (See Appendix II), (b) organization of structural components involved in actual administration of the service, (c) implementation of the training program, and (d) community liaison. However, what began as a crisis-intervention hotline rapidly evolved into an information and referral service because of problems such as conflict of interest with the university, the extent of responsibility assumed by paraprofessional volunteers, the restrictiveness of the service to the aging (as opposed to any-aged callers in crisis), and results of a need-assessment survey in which other crisis-intervention phone services were found to service the same community. Phase II of the project (unimplemented) was to have instituted outreach within a primary prevention model: paraprofessionals were to travel in pairs to the community and knock on doors. This strategy would have resolved one problem faced by hotline or information and referral phone services, in which callers fail to contact the service because of denial of problem, or simple unawareness of the existence of the service.

CONTINUUM OF CARE

In severe cases of physical or psychological disturbance, the nursing home or psychiatric institution may well provide the most appropriate setting. However, adequate supportive community services (e.g., home health care) could enable most aging persons to remain in their own homes. Where the family and the aging relative have reached mutual agreement about living together, day care could enable an extended-family situation to work. Represented along this continuum of care, as conceptualized by Rathbone-McCuan and Levenson (1975), would be (1) senior-citizen centers for individuals in average health and seeking a social situation where they can meet with peers, develop friends, and engage in activities to make life more meaningful, but who do not require custodial care and are not at risk for illness; and (2) day-care centers for individuals whose mental and/or physical health no longer enables them to remain in the community, who have no supportive family or surrogate family without which they would be at risk for total institutionalization.

Senior-citizen centers are perhaps the most well-known type of community service. The typical center consists of a group of healthy, well-motivated, active aging persons seeking social interaction. Private senior citizen's clubs are characterized by exclusivity and are not really open to any and all members, making this again a service unavailable to the impoverished aging person. State-run senior-citizen centers tend to provide more services, such as nutritional programs with hot lunches, routine health checkups, recreational programs. In addition, they include a trained staff with a number of paraprofessionals who can assist in making referrals, when necessary, and otherwise provide psychosocial intervention.

Day-treatment has attracted a great deal of attention, as well it should, yet there are surprisingly few of these essential programs in the United States today. Day-treatment centers generally provide transportation to and from the program, enabling the aging to continue to live at home, either alone or with family. They ensure a pleasant and supportive supervised environment with recreational activities and meals. Most importantly, they provide hospice services for the family. Social components of the program might include a beauty shop, religious activities, a library, field trips, music, and arts and crafts, to name but a few possibilities. Staffing for these centers can clearly tap paraprofessional resources on a full-time salaried basis. According to Rathbone-McCuan and Levenson (1975), "Day care centers are designed to provide services to aged persons with social role loss resulting from the combination of advanced age and functional disabilities."

Controversy over the target population to be served by geriatric day-treatment centers has greatly retarded their acceptance by the health community. One faction argues that day care should effectively replace existing community services and provide in-house health services as well. Such health services would include individualized psychological and medical intervention for those aging who suffer from disabilities, including prescribing medication, providing rehabilitation for physical (e.g., speech) handicaps, examinations, and testing. The other faction argues that day treatment should supplement existing community services, such as senior-citizen centers, and provide referrals where necessary. Thus, the former model envisions geriatric day care as a service for the physically or emotionally frail or infirm aging, whereas the latter views it as a means of serving the community aging at risk for, but currently suffering with, special physical or psychological problems (Weissert, 1976).

The first model is viewed as having positive features in that it services community aging who might otherwise need to be institutionalized, is well defined, but has negative features involving excessive costs. The second model is more cost effective but has negative features involving duplication of services already available through other community agencies. One could here argue the bête noire of short-term versus long-term cost effectiveness, and accountability to community versus state or federal funding agencies.

One proposed solution (Butler, 1979) has been to situate day-treatment centers within the environment of the total institution. There, medical and psychological rehabilitative services, including crisis-care capacity, would be available on-site where necessary, but not as a built-in requirement of the daily program. Another benefit of this model is that it provides an important transitional service for persons who are in the process of, or have recently been, discharged, but who could still derive benefit from the institution. Its apparent drawback is that it is perceived by the aging and the community as a form of institutionalization due to its physical location within the institutional environs.

General agreement has, however, been reached on the cost effectiveness of day-treatment versus multi-service or decentralized service provision (Hudson, 1974), in that it averts or postpones the need for total institutionalization. The basic core day-treatment program includes: (a) a daily program of social/recreational activities; (b) group intervention (e.g., milieu therapy) of some sort; (c) medication supervision, where necessary; (d) monthly monitoring of vital signs such as weight, pulse, blood pressure; (e) provision of hot noon meal; (f) negotiation, scheduling, and monitoring of health and social-service referrals; (g) education pertaining to aging health care, nutrition, Medicare/Medicaid, and SSI benefits; and (h) ongoing review through regular case conference and contact with family where available. Thus, the chief advantage of day-treatment is that it is flexible. An additional advantage of day-treatment is that the staff can consist largely of paraprofessionals who can implement many, if not all, of the above-mentioned service requirements.

"Adequacy and appropriateness of care is not guaranteed merely by not hospitalizing an old person, nor can good care be assured simply by the creation of geriatric screening teams, additional nursing homes and family care placements." (Markson, Levitz, and Gognalons-Caillard, 1973). What needs to be stressed is the fact that less than 5% of all aging persons are currently institutionalized, and a good proportion of these are probably unnecessarily institutionalized. Thus, home-delivered care, coordinated health maintenance, assistance with housekeeping, meals, transportation, health, and other essential services, and crisis intervention and counseling would be indicated for the category of community aging whose usual form of "intervention" are senior citizen's programs. For the other category of community aging who require some degree of assistance, the day-treatment center is one rational and sorely needed alternative.

Chapter 11

ADVOCACY

Mobilization Against Ageism

The thrust of any advocacy movement is the mobilization of members of special-interest groups to enable them to derive benefits from social and economic systems to which they are legitimately entitled, or to bring to bear sufficient political pressure to expand the provision of legislation to improve the quality of life for that group. In order to ensure that the special-interest group receives coordinated and quality services, there should be a single agency or person acting as agent or advocate with prime responsibility for seeing that these needs are met.

Advocates in grass-roots movements are beginning to be extremely effective in inducing social change. Nearly half of Florida's aging population, for example, belong to the American Association of Retired Persons or its parent organization, the National Teachers Association. Their lobbying has successfully resulted in a generic-drug law, consumer-advocacy agency, life-insurance reform, outlawing of unfair leasing practices, criminal-code revisions, increased public transportation, and more (Smith,

1979). Consciousness-raising groups such as the National Action Forum for Older Women and the Task Force of Older Women consist of advocates coordinated by social-science professionals working from the government (Administration on Aging) on down to the grass roots to combat ageism. Special-interest groups such as the Gray Panthers were built largely upon personal communication networks among politically active career women who were highly motivated by personal experience with job discrimination to form a coalition of advocates for the aging (Kuhn, 1975).

Advocacy movements actually preceded governmental interest in this special-interest group and grew in response to a particular sociocultural climate that made it possible to question previously accepted stereotypes about the aging. This climate, characterized by the affluence of the 1960s (when the plight of the underprivileged was being examined in part as a response to social conscience), was the same climate responsible for the rapid rise of the community mental-health movement in America. It is possible that the success of the anti-ageism movement (but not of the community mental-health movement) stems from the fact that grass-roots movements insure social change to a greater extent than movements whose motivators originate from without the organization.

The anti-ageism movement popularized by groups such as the Gray Panthers, combined with parallel movements toward deinstitutionalization, was then taken up by the Department of Health, Education and Welfare's Administration on Aging. Under the Older Americans Act, funding was provided to the state to allocate subarea support. One idea behind the Act was to remove sources of ageism along with individual and social barriers to independence, but this like many other community-health notions generally failed to be accomplished.

The health professions, following much the same pattern as the rest of American society in their attitudes toward the aging, have steadily discriminated against the aging client in theory and in treatment. Descriptive accounts of ageism in the health professions abound. Medical texts treat issues relating to the geriatric patient in an archaic and deprecatory manner (Breytspraak, 1978), and medical interns refer to aging patients as "crocks" (Butler and Lewis, 1973). Ageism is particularly visible in the area of attributing the diagnostic label "senile dementia" to instances of acute brain syndrome (Libow, 1973; Fox, Topel, and Huckman, 1975; Ernst, Badash, Beran, Kosovsky, and Kleinhauz, 1977; Settin, 1978), depression (Butler, 1975; Perlich and Atkins, 1979; Cavenar, Matbie, and Austin, 1979), or even normal behavior (Carp, 1969). The preferred clinical age group tends to be younger rather than older for nurses (Brown, 1967; Campbell, 1971), social workers (Mutschler, 1971), psychiatrists (Aronson and Weintraub, 1968; Cyrus-Lutz and Gaitz, 1972; Whanger and Busse, 1976), psychotherapists (Kastenbaum, 1964; Garfinkel, 1975; Settin, 1980), and gerontologists (Blank, 1978).

Ageism among health professionals is thus generally linked to an ideological orientation dominated by a medical stereotype of aging, where the geriatric client is seen as responsive only to custodial or palliative care (Coe, 1967), and by the theme of deterioration: "Medicine and the behavioral sciences have mirrored societal attitudes by presenting old age as a grim litany of physical and emotional ills. Decline of the individual has been the key concept" (Butler and Lewis, 1973).

Another example of "victim blaming" occurs when the aging are accused of avoiding contact with psychotherapists, when the objective reality is that psychotherapists avoid contact with them. Kastenbaum (1964) has proposed four explanations for the therapist's reluctance to treat the aging: (a) fear of one's own aging, (b) younger clients have longer to live, (c) association with depressed persons itself is found to be depressing, and (d) association with persons of low socioeconomic status (of which many aging typically are) is felt to be a contaminating element. The fourth explanation, that devalued persons such as the aging tend to be more unsatisfying for social status and economic reasons, has also been proposed by Rose and Peterson (1975).

Granick (1975) adds the explanation that: "It is difficult and uncomfortable for relatively young individuals to identify with and have empathy for the problems of an age level they have not personally experienced and which, in our culture, is regarded with negative and rejective reactions. Associated with this are prejudices about the lack of intellectual and personality effectiveness and resourcefulness in the aged which may generate feelings of potential boredom and hopelessness in the psychotherapist." The reluctant therapist is thus (a) status concerned, (b) lacking in direct experience with the aging, and (c) negatively biased toward the aging.

Recent systematic attempts to empirically quantify ageism in the health setting have resulted in confirmation of age discrimination. Kucharski, White, and Schratz (1979) mailed physicians a survey containing eight case histories describing both male and female, young and old stimulus patients. Results indicated that the symptomatology largely determined whether or not physicians showed age bias, which was measured by likelihood that physicians made referrals for psychological assistance. Perlich and Atkins (1979) presented 36 clinical psychologists working in state psychiatric hospitals with a taped interview of a depressed male of either 55 or 75 years of age. Dependent measures of diagnosis and severity of symptomatology resulted in age effect; when psychologists thought they were rating a 75-year-old, they were more likely to diagnose senile dementia than depression, and to give more severe judgments of "illness."

A national survey investigating client characteristics as determinants of clinical psychologists' perceptions of stimulus clients (Settin, 1979c) yielded strong evidence for age discrimination. In this survey, a case history containing one of eight possible combinations of the independent client characteristics of age (46/72), class (working/middle), and gender was sent, with follow-up prompts, to 800 randomly assigned American Psychological Association members. Components of perceptions, measured along a six-point Lichter scale "behavioral differential" were: (1) attitudes (statements about the client, tapping dependent variables: usefulness of intervention, prognosis, interest in providing intervention, comfort, likeability, competency, warmth, activity, strength, understandability); (2) symptom attribution, tapping dependent variables: disorientation, egocentricism, hypochondrosis, impaired judgment, inadequate hygiene, inappropriate behavior, incoherent speech, intolerance for change, reminiscence, stereotyped behavior, suspiciousness, thought disorder; and (3) diagnosis. The final sample of 418 respondents returned data that were analyzed with a Multivariate Analysis of Variance, demonstrating that the 72-year-old client elicited significantly more severe pathology according to assigned diagnosis (e.g., "psychosis"), attributed symptomology (e.g., "disorientation"), and expression of negative attitude (e.g., "usefulness of intervention") than did the 46-year-old client. This tendency of clinical psychologists to perceive aging clients as more deviant based upon an age label alone provides empirical evidence for the existence of ageism in the health setting.

Recent mobilization of health professionals against ageism, in combination with a growing grass-roots movement led by community advocates for the aging, serves as a visible testimony that social change is occurring. Much of this change has been accomplished through public education involving dissemination of correct factual information about the aging process. The willingness of funding agencies to support innovative new roles for paraprofessionals in gerontology will be largely determined by the degree to which ageism diminishes and the speed with which attitude change accelerates. At present, one area in which health paraprofessionals can have considerable impact toward combating ageism and assisting the aging in obtaining equal rights is demythologizing aging.

PROVISION OF INDIRECT SERVICES

Areas of concentration for the community-aging advocate, who functions primarily as a community resource person relying heavily on information and referral services, are: (1) analysis of health-delivery systems in terms of their purpose, mandate, and structure, (2) development of appropriate models for health-care delivery, (3) investigation of community and system resources available for health-care delivery, (4) evaluation of the role of the paraprofessional advocate within the health-care system, (5) relationship of recommendations for enhancement of health-care delivery to the paraprofessional role, (6) understanding the political, legal, and economic realities of advocacy, and (7) prevention of client victimization.

An information-giving service of the community advocate would be provision of correct factual information concerning the process of normal aging. Clients receiving public education will be better able to evaluate their behavior in relation to societal expectations. Many aging persons are laboring under the misapprehension that their problems are due to a personal failure, or that there is little hope for their future. Through the use of relaxed, nonevaluative seminars, the aging advocate can disseminate information in a variety of pre-existing supportive environments such as the church, school system (continuing education for adults), and other civic associations.

Providing linkages to community networks and understanding the basic structure of community systems well enough to be able to build a community referral network through contacts is an important part of the advocate's role. A referral should reflect the most direct route the aging client can take in order to obtain what is needed. The paraprofessional will need to evaluate the source of the referral (e.g., where did the paraprofessional hear about this service, is it reliable, and so on) to ensure that the client actually will be receiving the recommended service once referral is accomplished. For example, the senior-citizen center listed in the county's social-services manual may no longer be in operation, the phone number may have changed, or there may be restrictions for membership.

Because of differences in socialization and life experience, the aging may not be skilled in stating their needs and asserting their rights, and may be intimidated by bureaucratic red tape. Since the aging, like "low-income people require the concrete services of some of these systems for sheer survival as well as for their social and psychological well being, their inability to voice their needs effectively contributes to their sense of powerlessness, anomie and frustration and reinforces their self-defeating behavior" (Peck, Kaplan, and Roman, 1965). These people need an advocate to help them actively deal with problems with social service, health care, and business agencies that are used to dealing through intermediaries. They have distinct approach patterns with which younger persons are familiar but with which aging persons are not. Bureaucracies also speak a language all their own, making transactions of the simplest sort almost unintelligible to the uninitiated. An example would be obtaining a personal loan from a bank, and having to wade through "bankese" involving "makers," equities, prepayment penalties, deferred interest rates, and so on.

Of all the areas in which the aging need strong advocacy, employment is in the forefront. There is growing pressure being applied to obtain volunteer and paid supplementary jobs for the aging who cannot make do with small pensions, Social Security, and the increasing costs of home maintenance. For example, an active advocate with the National Committee on Careers for Older Americans proposed that counseling and training services needed to match people and jobs in conjunction with "vocational schools, community colleges and public and private employment agencies and labor organizations" would to "work together to identify existing jobs or prospective jobs that could be filled by aging persons" (Flemming, 1979).

Additional objectives of the paraprofessional aging advocate are to assist in identifying significant economic, cultural, psychosocial, and environmental determinants of health problems in aging, and to assist in analysis of these needs of community aging. In pursuit of these objectives, paraprofessionals may participate in community-based evaluation research emphasizing the interaction of networks of health-care delivery systems. Moos (1973) has proposed a useful paradigm for the facilitation and evaluation of mobilization in groups having high amounts of interaction among their members. This paradigm, which could be introduced by paraprofessionals within total institutions on wards or community settings in senior citizen centers, includes assessment, feedback, planning, and reassessment.

More specifically, a senior-citizen group is concerned with victimization of the aging in their community by absentee landlords. The paraprofessional, acting as advocate for the group, guides the group through (a) evaluation of the problem: a "man-on-the-street survey is carried out to collect information about the aging involved in the problem, (b) feedback, which is given to the aging in the community through leaflet, newsletter, and newspaper article about who the victims are (demographic data), (c) an open-to-the-community planning meeting, where the citizens group, now serving as advocate for other community aging, proposes a course of action to deal with the problem and carry out the proposed intervention, and (d) reassessment, performed to evaluate the effectiveness of the program in reducing victimization.

In addition to indirect services, such as information and referral, the allied-health paraprofessional will be providing direct services to the aging in a caseworker format. Case-management functions would involve therapeutic intervention, including interviewing and feedback of findings to the aging client, testing and crisis-in-intervention services. These direct community services do not differ substantially from previously discussed institutional services for the aging.

ETHICAL AND LEGAL RESPONSIBILITIES

Paraprofessionals working in the field of aging are required to be thoroughly familiar with guidelines to ethical behavior with clients, and with legal regulations that directly influence the clients' well-being. It is now a routine practice to furnish all clients with a "bill of rights" upon admission to hospitals, clinics or nursing homes, and to inform them periodically of changes in policy concerning the voluntariness of their status or facility policy otherwise applicable.

The problem with this is that regulations are not always easy to understand and the client may sign papers that bear on the disposal of personal property, too late comprehending the implications. Further, the distinction between competency and incompetency as it relates to comprehension of legal language is hazy. There is also the clause granting right to refuse treatment. This clause, introduced to eliminate over-restrictive treatment for a client who is sufficiently recovered to be ready for discharge, sometimes results in the situation where the client is receiving no medication (if refused), attending no organized activities, and generally failing to benefit from the resources of the institution, thereby ensuring continued institutionalization.

Signing a bill of rights does not ensure that informal interactions between staff and client will proceed ethically. This is not to imply that unethical activities are performed with malice of forethought, but rather that certain situations may be handled carelessly through ignorance or insensitivity. It is the paraprofessional's responsibility to accord clients every consideration possible that does not interfere with what is deemed by the whole treatment team to be therapeutic intervention. What is deemed therapeutic by some may not seem so to others, and this is an ongoing debate in health care; it is for this reason that treatment-team consultations are vital.

Staff become "institutionalized" just as easily as do clients. They may hear professionals talking about clients right in front of the client and think that this is a normal and correct thing to do. They may have been in the same job for so long that they become apathetic from lack of reinforcement, poor working conditions, or boredom. They may have found their own attempts at change frustrated by other staff or by policy restrictions, and may have tried and failed at interventions and as a result may resent attempts of others to initiate treatment programs. Or they may just not like their job and be due for a change. Whatever the reason, there is never any excuse for unethical behavior in front of a client. The paraprofessional can go home at the end of the day—the client cannot. The four examples of unethical behavior that follow are commonly observed and are cited because they could make the difference between the competent paraprofessional and someone who should not be working in a clinical setting.

Treating the Client as an Object

This simulated conversation between two staff persons (with the client standing by) devalues the client by talking about her as if she were an inanimate object and by disparaging her capabilities. Notice how the one staff person shows sensitivity to the situation by requesting that the conversation continue in private, by including the client in the remainder of conversation, and by making a positive statement to encourage the client in the face of negative reinforcement.

S1: I'm going to spend a few minutes with Ms. T. to work on her verbal skills.

S2: It won't do you any good.

S1: What do you mean?

S2: She hasn't said a word for years and nobody else here has had any luck with her so I don't see why you would.

S1: Do you think we could talk about this in private?

S2: We're private here—nobody's listening.

S1: Well, Ms. T. is listening.

S2: Oh, that doesn't matter—she can't understand half of it.

S1: (turning to include Ms. T. in conversation) Ms. T. said a few words to me the other day and that was very encouraging. The speech therapist says that there is nothing wrong with her ability to speak, but that she hardly knows any English, right Ms. T.?

S2: (with obvious disbelief) Humph. Good luck.

S1: Thank you. Let's go, Ms. T.

Overstepping Responsibility

Overstepping responsibility happens to everyone sooner or later, and it is a safe policy to spend the first several weeks in any new setting listening a lot and keeping most of one's opinions to oneself. Overstepping responsibility can result in serious consequences for the paraprofessional, the client, and the facility. An example would be a client who is waiting for a transfer out of a nursing home. The client tells the paraprofessional that the professional staff isn't doing anything about getting the transfer. When the paraprofessional tactfully asks the professional about it, message is that everything is being done as quickly as possible. Not believing this the paraprofessional goes ahead and initiates a transfer contact with another facility. This results in bad staff relations, and is unethical behavior on the paraprofessional's part. Firstly, there is no clear evidence that the professional is being negligent; secondly, the paraprofessional has no training in referral; thirdly, the paraprofessional is going over the professional's head. The person who suffers the most for this is the client, who is now blamed for causing trouble and is denied transfer.

Release of Unauthorized Information

It is often the case that the paraprofessional has more family contact than the professional, and may in fact "know" the client better. The family comes in to visit and asks the paraprofessional how the client is doing. The client's chart shows a very poor prognosis, but the clinician in charge has not yet informed the family. Nonetheless, the paraprofessional gently breaks the news, the family members become upset and call the physician on emergency to demand to know why they weren't informed of this sudden change in the client's condition. No matter how much the paraprofessional knows about a case, no matter how sure that "this is exactly what the physician would have said," no matter how much the family pleads for information, there is no excuse for

releasing information about a client's condition until the professional gives direct orders that it may be done. Alternately, imagine
the paraprofessional who tells the family that the client seems to be
improving. A few hours later, the client dies. This is even worse,
yet it happens all the time.

Violation of Confidentiality

A client has confided to the paraprofessional that he left the
facility the other day without permission and went to town. He
asks that no one be told and the paraprofessional consents. In
talking with a co-worker, the paraprofessional relates the incident
and then says "but don't tell anyone." The next day, the client is
grounded for a week. The paraprofessional has behaved unethical-
ly by using the client's privileged information as a topic of conversation, and has betrayed the confidence and trust that had been
established between the client and paraprofessional. Confidentiality is as inviolate and privileged as information given to a priest at
confessional. If confidentiality is broken, there had better be a
good reason. For example, if the client in question were a diabetic
and had left the facility to have an ice cream soda with plenty of
sugar that could bring on an insulin reaction, it would be important
to record this information for purposes of the client's health in the
chart. In this event, the paraprofessional should not promise the
client confidentiality and should explain why.

One final note of caution: although it is highly unlikely that
the paraprofessional would become personally involved with an
aging client in a romantic or sexual way, suffice it to say that this is
a nontherapeutic relationship for the client and under no circumstances is it acceptable to do so.

Legal repercussions can result from unethical behavior, and
while many of these guidelines are spelled out, others that involve
personal judgment are less explicit and open to interpretation. In
general, should there be any questions about a procedure, the best
policy is to ask. Legal action is most likely to follow from unethical behavior or alleged unethical behavior that touches upon some

taboo, such as sex, drug abuse, or brutality. Others are neglecting to report hazardous conditions, ignoring an emergency, performing unauthorized medical services, theft, and releasing unauthorized information.

In recent years there have been several controversial lawsuits brought against staff for applying physical restraint to a client who is "deemed to be dangerous to himself or to others." It is obviously both unethical and illegal to use restraint except under certain circumstances; however, the interpretation of "dangerous" is open to question and depends on a number of variables. For example, a client who actually is becoming uncontrollably violent and attacks the paraprofessional might be responded to with the normal reaction of trying to ward off injury. Afterward, the client could charge that unlawful restraint was employed, and there may have been no witnesses, resulting in an inquest. There are proper and improper methods of restraint. Those that are not under any circumstances damaging to the client should be learned by paraprofessionals if they are going to be working with assaultive populations.

In the community setting, paraprofessionals working as advocates in direct service may encounter problems with ethics of the intervention itself (e.g., is it a therapeutically or educationally oriented activity?). A second and more fundamental issue is the privilege of persons to be left to their own beliefs. The client will often be operating with a set of convictions rooted in radically different morality or politicality than that of the paraprofessional. In indirect service, it is even more difficult to determine to what extent the process treated in the intervention involves other persons and in what capacity they will be affected. Thus, the paraprofessional actually has the capability to wield power over the client and other unwitting individuals, and as a result careful examination of the paraprofessional's motives in recommending certain courses of action should take place.

Specifically, mental-health intervention agents can use their power to control deviant behavior (Lemert, 1967). It is unconscionable for the power holder (the advocate) to put personal goals above the goals of the client. Since it is simply not possible to operate as a value-free agent, the issue is not whether the advocates introject their own value systems into the intervention process, but to what extent and by what means. Health-care delivery systems are now becoming deeply concerned with appropriateness, accountability, and ethicality because they are being subjected to increasing scrutiny. Accrediting committees abound, almost to the point of creating unmanageable amounts of paperwork that could eventually interfere with performance. Despite this, further checks and balances are needed, as advocacy is in its infancy.

REFERENCES

Appleby, T. W. Evaluation of treatment methods for chronic schizophrenia. *Archives of General Psychiatry,* 1963, *8,* 8–21.

Arenberg, D. Cognition and aging: Verbal learning, memory, and problem solving. *Psychology of adult development and aging,* 1973, 74–97.

Aronson, H., and Weintraub, W. Social background of the patient in classical psychoanalysis. *Journal of Nervous and Mental Disease,* 1968, *146,* 91–97.

Atthowe, J. M. Controlling nocturnal enuresis in severely disabled and chronic patients. *Behavior Therapy,* 1972, *3,* 232–239.

Barker, R. G. *Ecological psychology,* Stanford, California: Stanford University Press, 1968.

Barnes, E. K., Sack, A., and Shore, H. Guidelines to treatment approaches. *The Gerontologist,* 1973, *13,* 513–527.

Becker, W., and Cesar, J. A. Use of beer in geriatric psychiatric patient groups. *Psychological Reports,* 1973, *33*(1), 182.

Bell, B. D. Mobile medical care to the elderly: An evaluation. *The Gerontologist,* 1975, *15,* 100–103.

Bell, W. G. Community care for the elderly: An alternative to institutionalization. *The Gerontologist, 1973,* Autumn, Part I, 329–354.

Bellucci, G., and Hoyer, W. J. Feedback effects on the performance and self-reinforcing behavior of elderly and young adult women. *Journal of Gerontology,* 1975, *30*(4), 456–460.

Benjamin, A. *The helping interview*. Boston, Massachusetts: Houghton Mifflin Co., 1974.

Bergin, A. E., and Soloman, S. *Personality and performance correlates of empathic understanding in psychology*. Paper presented at annual meeting of the American Psychological Association, Philadelphia, Pennsylvania, September 1963.

Berg, W. E., Atlas, L., and Zeiger, J. Integrated homemaking services for the aged in urban neighborhoods. *The Gerontologist*, 1974, *14*.

Bierman, E. L., and Brody, H. (Chairs), *Our future selves*. Report of the Panel on Biomedical Research. DHEW Publ. No. (NIH) 78–1445, 1976.

Birjani, P. F., and Sclafani, M. J. An interdisciplinary team approach to geriatric patient care. *Hospital and Community Psychiatry*, 1973, *24*(11), 777–778.

Birkett, D. P., and Boltuch, B. Remotivation therapy. *Journal of the American Geriatrics Society*, 1973, *21*, 368–371.

Birren, J. *The psychology of aging*. Englewood Cliffs, New Jersey: Prentice-Hall, 1964.

Birren, J. J., and Renner, V. J. *Stress and aging: Psychobiological theory and research*. Paper presented at Gerontological Society Meeting, New York, New York, October 1976.

Blank, M. L. *Ageism in gerontologyland*. Paper presented at 31st Annual Meeting of the Gerontological Society, Dallas, Texas, 1978.

Blau, Z. S. *Old age in a changing society*. New York: New Viewpoints, 1973.

Braginsky, B. *The Dynamics of Expendability: Studies in the Abbreviation of Man*. Unpublished manuscript, 1978.

Breytspraak, L. M. *Medical texts as sources of physician attitudes toward the geriatric patient*. Paper presented at 31st Annual Meeting of the Gerontological Society, Dallas Texas, 1978.

Brill, H. (principal investigator), A study of the role of state and area agencies on aging in the provision of common support services for deinstitutionalized elderly mental health patients and the non-institutionalized vulnerable elderly. New York: Health Systems Planning Foundation of Suffolk, 1979.

Brocklehurst, J. E. Recent advances in incontinence. In G. Judge (Ed.), *Geriatric medicine*, New York: Academic Press, 1974.

Brody, H. Structural changes in the aging nervous system. *Interdisciplinary topics in gerontology*, Volume 7. New York: Karger-Munchen, 1970.

Brown, M. I. *Nursing Care of the Aged*. In F. Jeffers (Ed.), Proceedings of seminars 1965–69, Duke University Council on Aging and Human Development. Durham, North Carolina: Duke University Medical Center, 1969.

Brubaker, T. H., and Powers, E. A. The stereotype of old: A review and alternative approach. *Journal of Gerontology*, 1976, *31*(4) 441–447.

Buckley, C. E., III, and Dorsey, F. C. Serum immunoglobulin concentrations. *Journal of Immunology*, 1970, *105*(4), 964–972.

Burnside, I. M. Group work with the aged: Selected literature. *The Gerontologist,* 1970, *10*(3, 1), 241–246.

Burnside, I. M. Touching is talking. *American Journal of Nursing,* 1973, *73*(12), 2060–2063.

Busse, E. M. *Therapeutic implications of basic research with the aging.* Strecker monograph series No. IV, University of Pennsylvania Hospital, Philadelphia, Pennsylvania, 1967.

Busse, E. W. Organic brain syndromes. In E. W. Busse and E. Pfeiffer (Eds.), *Mental Illness in Later Life,* Washington, D.C.: APA Publications, 1973.

Busse, E. W., and Pfeiffer, E. Functional psychiatric disorders in old age. In E. W. Busse and E. Pfeiffer (Eds.), *Behavior and adaptation in late life,* Boston, Massachusetts: Little, Brown & Co., 1969.

Butler, R. N. *The elderly person with mental health problems - "Is it a closed door?"* Address presented at workshop, Central Islip Psychiatric Center, Central Islip, New York: October 5, 1979.

Butler, R. N. Age-ism: Another form of bigotry. *The Gerontologist,* 1969, *9,* 243–246.

Butler, R. N. *Why survive? Being old in America.* New York: Harper & Row Publications, 1975.

Butler, R. N., and Lewis, M. I. *Aging and mental health: Positive psychological approaches.* St. Louis, Missouri: C. V. Morby, 1973.

Butler, R. N., Dastur, D. K., and Perlin, S. Relationships of senile manifestations and chronic brain syndromes to cerebral circulation and metabolism. *Journal of Psychiatric Research,* 1965, *3,* 229–238.

Calhoun, J. B. Population density and social pathology. *Scientific American,* 1962, *206,* 139–148.

Campbell, M. E. Study of the attitudes of nursing personnel toward the geriatric patient. *Nursing Research,* 1971, *20,* 147–151.

Caplan, G. *Principles of community psychiatry.* London: Tavistock Publications, 1964.

Caplow-Lindner, E., Harpaz, L., and Samberg, S. *Therapeutic dance movement: Expressive activities for older adults.* New York: Human Sciences Press, 1979.

Carkhuff, R. R. *Helping and human relations.* New York: Holt, Rinehart & Winston, 1969.

Carkhuff, R. R., and Traux, C. B. Lay mental health counseling: The effects of lay group counseling. *Journal of Consulting Psychology,* 1965, *29,* 426–431.

Carp, F. M. Senility or garden variety maladjustment? *Journal of Gerontology,* 1969, *24,* 203–208.

Cautela, J. R. Manipulation of the psychosocial environment of the geriatric patient. In Kent, Kastenbaum and Sherwood (Eds.), *Research planning and action for the elderly.* New York: Behavioral Publications, 1972.

Cavenar, J. O., Matbie, A. A., and Austin, L. Depression simulating OBD. *American Journal of Psychiatry*, 1979, *136*, 4B, 521–523.

Chien, C. Psychiatric treatment for geriatric patients: "Pub" or drug? *American Journal of Psychiatry*, 1971, *127*(8), 1070–1075.

Citrin, R. S., and Dixon, D. N. *Reality orientation: A milieu therapy used in an institution for the aged*. Paper presented at the Annual Meeting of the Gerontological Society, Louisville, Kentucky, October 1975.

Coe, R. M. Professional perspectives on the aged. *The Gerontologist*, 1967, *7*, 114–119.

Cohen, R. G. Outreach and advocacy in the treatment of the aged. *Social Casework*, 1974, *55*, 271–277.

Comstock, R. L., Mayers, R. L., and Folsom, J. C. Simple physical activities for the elderly. *Hospital and Community Psychiatry*, 1969, *20*, 377–380.

Cook, F. L., Skogan, W. G., Cook, T. D., and Antunes, G. E. Criminal victimization of the elderly: The physical and economic consequences. *The Gerontologist*, 1978, *18*(4), 338–349.

Corman, J. C. Health services for the elderly. In B. Neugarten and R. Havighurst (Eds.), *Social policy, social ethics and the aging society*. Washington, D.C.: U.S. Government Printing Office, 1973.

Cowen, E. I., Liebowitz, E. and Liebowitz, G. The utilization of retired people as mental health aides in the schools. *American Journal of Orthopsychiatry*, 1968, *38*, 900–909.

Crouch, D. D. Lighting needs for older eyes. *Journal of the American Geriatrics Society*, 1967, *15*, 684–688.

Cyrus-Lutz, C., and Gaitz, C. M. Psychiatrists' attitudes toward the aged and aging. *The Gerontologist*, 1972, *12*, 163–174.

Danish, S. J., and Augelli, A. R. rationale and implementation of a training program for paraprofessionals. *Professional Psychology*, 1976, *7*, 38–46.

Danish, S. J., and Hauer, A. E. *Helping skills: A basic training program*. New York: Behavioral Publications, 1973.

Davis, G. E., and Baum, A. *The role of architecturally determined loci of interaction in the development of residential communities*. Paper presented at meeting of American Psychological Association, Chicago, Illinois, September 2, 1975.

Dekker, E., and Groen, J. Reproducible psychogenic attacks of asthma. *Journal of Psychosomatic Research*, 1956, *1*, 58–67.

Dewdney, I. An art therapy program for geriatric patients. *American Journal of Art Therapy*, 1973, *12*(4), 249–254.

Donahue, W. T. *Older American Reports*, November 23, 1977, p. 6.

Dubey, E. Intensive treatment of the institutionalized, ambulatory geriatric patient. *Geriatrics*, 1968, *23*(6), 1970–178.

Durlak, J. A. Myths concerning the nonprofessional therapist. *Professional Psychology*, 1973, *4*, 300–304.

Eisdorfer, C. Some variables relating to longevity in humans. In A. M. Ostfeld and D. C. Gibson (Eds.), *Epidemiology of Aging*, DHEW Publications # (HEW) 75–711, 1972.

Eisdorfer, C., Nowlin, J., and Wilkie, F. Improvement of verbal learning in the aged by modification of autonomic nervous system activity. *Science*, 1970, *170*, 1327–1329.

Eisdorfer, C., and Wilkie, F. Auditory changes. *Journal of the American Geriatric Society*, 1972, *20*, 377–382.

Ellsworth, R. B. *Nonprofessionals in psychiatric rehabilitation*. New York: Appleton-Century-Crofts, 1968.

Ernst, P., Badash, D., Beran, B., Kosovsky, R., and Kleinberg, M. Incidence of mental illness in the aged: Unmasking the effects of a diagnosis of Chronic Brain Syndrome. *Journal of the American Geriatrics Society*, 1977, *25*(8), 371–375.

Exton-Smith, A. N. Vitamins and the elderly. In Anderson and Judge (Eds.), *Geriatric medicine*. New York: Academic Press, 1974.

Feifel, H. Attitudes toward death in some normal and mentally ill populations. In H. Feifel (Ed.), *The meaning of death*, New York: McGraw-Hill, 1959.

Feifel, H. The taboo of death. *American Behavioral Scientist*, 1963, *6*, 66–67.

Flemming, A. S. *Older Americans: An Untapped Resource*. Washington, D.C.: National Committee on Careers for Older Americans, 1979.

Fiske, M. *Symposium on Chronic Brain Syndromes*, annual meeting of Gerontological Society, New York, New York, October 1976.

Foley, J. M. Differential Diagnosis of Mental Disorders. In C. M. Gaitz (Ed.), *Aging and the brain*. New York: Plenum Press, 1972.

Ford, A. B. Distinguishing characteristics of the aging from a clinical viewpoint. *Journal of the American Geriatric Society*, 1968, *16*(1), 142–148.

Fox, J. H., Topel, J. L., and Huckman, M. S. Dementia in the elderly—A search for treatable illnesses. *Journal of Gerontology*, 1975 *30*(5), 557–564.

Gaitz, C. M., and Baer, P. E. Characteristics of eldery patients with alcoholism. *Archives of General Psychiatry*, 1971, *24*, 372–378.

Gardner, E., Bahn, A. K., and Mack, M. Suicide and psychiatric care in the aging. *Archives of General Psychiatry*, 1963, *10*, 547–553.

Garfinkel, R. The reluctant therapist 1975. *The Gerontologist*, 1975, *15*(2), 136–137.

Geiger, O. G., and Johnson, L. A. Positive education for elderly persons: Correct eating through reinforcement. *The Gerontologist*, 1974, *14*, 422,–436.

Goffman, E. *Asylums: Essays on the social situation of mental patients and other inmates*. New York: Anchor Books, 1961.

Gottesman, L. E. The response of long hospitalized aged psychiatric patients to milieu treatment. *The Gerontologist*, 1967, *7*(1), 47–48.

Goldfried, M. R., and Davison, G. C. *Clinical behavior therapy*. New York: Holt, Rinehart & Winston, 1976.

Goldstein, S. A critical appraisal of milieu therapy in a geriatric day hospital. *Journal of the American Geriatric Society*, 1971, *19*, 693–699.

Goodman, G. Systematic selection of therapeutic talent: The group assessment of interpersonal traits. In S. E. Golann and C. Eisdorfer (Eds.), *Handbook of community mental health*. New York: Appleton-Century-Crofts, 1972.

Gordon, J. E. Project cause, the federal anti-poverty program and some implications of subprofessional training. *American Psychologist*, 1965, 30, 334–343.

Gove, W. R. Societal reaction as an explanation of mental illness: An evaluation. *American Sociological Review*, 1970, *35*, 873–884.

Granick, S. *Group and family therapies with the aged*. Paper presented at Symposium on Psychotherapy with the Aged, Annual Meeting American Psychological Association, September 1975, Chicago, Illinois.

Granick, S., and Patterson, R. D. *Human Aging II: An 11 Year Follow-Up Biomedical and Behavioral Study*. U.S. Department of Government Printing Office, 1971.

Gruman, G. J. Cultural Origins of present-day "age-ism": The modernization of the life cycle. In S. F. Spicker, K. M. Woodward, and D. D. Van Tassel (Eds.), *Aging and the elderly: Human perspectives in gerontology*. Atlantic Highlands, New Jersey: Humanities Press, 1978.

Gurian, B. S., and Scherl, D. J. A community-focused model of mental health services for the eldery. *Journal of Geriatric Psychiatry*, 1972, *5*(1), 77–86.

Haase, G. R. Diseases presenting as dementia. *Contemporary Neurology*, 1971, *9*, 163–207.

Hallowitz, E., and Reissman, F. The role of the indigenous nonprofessional in a community mental health neighborhood service center program. *American Journal of Orthopsychiatry*, 1967, *37*, 766–778.

Harris, L., and Associates, Inc. *The myth and reality of aging in America*. National Council on the Aging, Inc. Washington, D.C., 1975, 46–55.

Haskell, M. *The new careers concept: Potential for public employment of the poor*. New York: Praeger Publications, 1969.

Hellerstein, H. E. Heart disease and sex. *Medical Aspects of Human Sexuality*, 1971, *5*(6), 24–35.

Hickey, T. Training for a supportive geriatric environment: A preliminary report. *Journal of Community Psychology*, 1976, *4*, 261–268.

Hickey, T. Simulating age-related sensory impairments for practitioner education. *The Gerontologist*, 1975, *15*(5,1), 457–463.

Honigfeld, G., and Klett, C. J. The nurses' observation scale for inpatient evaluation. *Journal of Clinical Psychology*, 1965, *21*, 65–71.

Hoyer, W. J., Kafer, R. A., Simpson, S. C., and Hoyer, F, W. Reinstatement of verbal behavior in elderly mental patients using operant procedures. *The Gerontologist*, 1974, *14*, 149–152.

Hoyer, W. T., Labouvie, G. V., and Baltes, P. B. Modification of response speed deficits and intellectual performance in the elderly. *Human Development*, 1973, *16*, 233–242.

Hoyer, W. J., Mishara, B. L., and Riebel, R. G. Problem behaviors as operants: Applications with elderly individuals. *The Gerontologist*, 1975, *15*(5,1), 452–456.

Hudson, E. M. day care center cost effectiveness analysis: Preliminary Report. New York: Community Research Applications, Inc., 1974.

Jarvik, L. F., and Cohen, D. A biobehavioral approach to intellectual changes with aging. *Psychology of adult development and aging*, 1973, 220–280.

Jeffers, F. C., Nichols, C. R., and Eisdorfer, C. Attitudes of older persons toward death: A preliminary study. *Journal of Gerontology*, 1961, *16*, 53–56.

Jeger, A. M. *Training nonprofessional behavior change agents: A review of the literature*. Unpublished manuscript, State University of New York, Stony Brook, 1976.

Jones, M. *The therapeutic community*. New York: Basic Books, 1953.

Judge, T. G. Nutrition in the elderly. *Geriatric Medicine*, 1974, 231–245.

Kahana, E., Liang, J., Felton, B., Fairchild, B., and Harel, Z. Perspectives of aged on victimization, "ageism," and their problems in urban society. *The Gerontologist*, 1977, *17*(2), 121–129.

Kahn, R. L. The mental health system and the future aged. *The Gerontologist*, 1975, *15*, 24–31.

Kastenbaum, R. Perspective on the development and modification of behavior in the aged: A developmental—field perspective. *The Gerontologist*, 1968, *8*, 280–283.

Kastenbaum, R. The reluctant therapist. In R. K. Kastenbaum (Ed.), *New thoughts on old age*. New York: Springer Publishing Company, Inc., 1964.

Kastenbaum, R. and Aisenberg, R. *The psychology of death*. New York: Springer Publishing Company, 1976.

Katz, S., Ford, A. B., Maskowitz, R. W., Jackson, B. A., and Jaffe, M. W. Studies of illness in the aged. *Journal of the American Medical Association*, *185*(12), 1963.

Kennedy, R. D. Recent advances in cardiology. In Judge (Ed.), *Geriatric medicine*. New York: Academic Press, 1974.

Kirby, M. W., Polak, P., and Deever, S. *Community social environments versus psychiatric hospitalization: A research study*. Paper presented at American Psychological Association, Chicago, Illinois, September 2, 1975.

Kübler-Ross, E. *Death: The Final Stage of Growth*. Englewood Cliffs, New Jersey: Prentice-Hall, Inc., 1975.

Kucharski, L. J., White, R. M., and Schratz, M. Age bias, referral for psychological assistance and the private physician. *Journal of Gerontology*, 1971, *34*(3), 423–428.

Kuhn, M. Gray Panther power. *The Center Magazine*, 1975, *8*(2), 21–25.

Kushler, M. G., and Davidson, W. S. II. Alternative modes of outreach: An experimental comparison. *The Gerontologist,* 1978, *18* (4) 355–362.

Langer, E. J., and Abelson, R. P. A patient by any other name . . . : Clinician group differences in labeling bias. *Journal of Consulting and Clinical Psychology,* 1974, *42,* 4–9.

Lawton, M. P., Brody, E., and Turner-Massey, P. *The relationships of environmental factors to changes in well-being.* Paper presented at Symposium on Intermediate Housing for the Elderly. Annual meeting of Gerontological Society, New York, October 1976.

Lawton, M. P., Liebowitz, B., and Charon, H. Physical structure and the behavior of senile patients following ward remodeling. *Aging and Human Development,* 1970, *3*(1), 231–239.

Lemert, E. *Human deviance, social problems and social control.* Englewood Cliffs, New Jersey: Prentice-Hall, 1967.

Lewin, K. *Field theory in social science.* New York: Harper & Row, 1951.

Libow, L. S. Pseudo-senility: Acute and reversible organic brain syndromes. *Journal of the American Geriatric Society,* 1973, *21*(3), 112–120.

Liederman, P. C., Green, R., and Liederman, V. R. Outpatient group therapy with geriatric patients. *Geriatrics,* 1967, *22,* 148–153.

Lindsley, O. R. Geriatric behavioral prosthetics. In R. Kastenbaum (Ed.), *New thoughts on old age.* New York: Springer Publishing Company, 1964.

Lipman, A., and Slater, R. Homes for old people: Toward a positive environment. *The Gerontologist,* 1977, *17*(2), 146–156.

Lowenthal, M. F. The relationship between social factors and mental health in the aged. *Psychiatric Research Reports,* 1968, *23,* 187–197.

MacDonald, M. L. The forgotten Americans: A sociopsychological analysis of aging and nursing homes. *American Journal of Community Psychology,* 1973, *1,* 272–294.

MacDonald, M. L. Environmental programming for the socially isolated aging. *The Gerontologist,* 1978, *18*(4), 350–35.

MacDonald, M. L., and Butler, A. K. Reversal of helplessness: Producing walking behavior in nursing home wheelchair residents using behavior modification. *Journal of Gerontology,* 1973, *29,* 97–101.

MacDonald, M. L., and Settin, J. M. Reality orientation versus sheltered workshops as treatment for the institutionalized aging. *Journal of Gerontology,* 1978, *33*(3), 416–421.

Maier, S. F., and Seligman, M. E. P. Learned helplessness: Theory and evidence. *Journal of Experimental Psychology: General,* 1976, *105,* 3–46.

Markson, E. W., Levitz, F. S., and Gognalons-Caillard, M. The elderly and the community: Reidentifying unmet needs. *Journal of Gerontology,* 1973, *28*(4), 503–509.

Martin, J. D. Power, dependence, and the complaints of the elderly: A social exchange perspective. *Aging and Human Development,* 1971, *2*(2), 108–112.

Marx, A. J., Test, M. A., and Stein, L. I. Exohospital management of severe mental illness. *Archives of General Psychiatry,* 1973, *29,* 505–511.

McCluskey, N. G. Demographic profile of America's elderly. In CASE Center for Gerontological Studies Newsletter, *Catching Up on Aging,* 1978, *6.*

McClannahan, L. E., and Risley, T. R. Design of living environments for nursing home residents: Increasing participation in recreation activities. *Journal of Applied Behavior Analysis,* 1975, *8,* 261–268.

McTavish, D. G. Perceptions of old people. A review of research methodologies and findings. *The Gerontologist,* 1971, *11*(4), Part 2, 90–101.

Mechanic, D. *Mental health and social policy.* Englewood Cliffs, New Jersey: Prentice-Hall, 1969.

Meeker, R. A. *Utilization of preventive health services by the elderly.* Paper presented at 29th Annual Meeting of Gerontological Society, New York, New York: October 13–17, 1976.

Meichenbaum, D. The effects of instructions and reinforcement on thinking and language behavior of schizophrenics. *Behavior Research and Therapy,* 1969, *7,* 101–114.

Meichenbaum, D. Self-instructional strategy training: A cognitive prosthesis for the aged. *Human Development,* 1974, *17,* 273–280.

Meichenbaum, D., and Cameron, R. Training schizophrenics to talk to themselves: A means of developing attentional controls. *Behavior Therapy,* 1973, *4,* 515–534.

Mendel, W. M., and Rapport, S. Outpatient treatment for chronic schizophrenic patients: Therapeutic consequences of an existential view. *Archives of General Psychiatry,* 1963, *8,* (2), 190–196.

Merton, R. K. *Social theory and social structure.* Glencoe, New York: The Free Press, 1957.

Mezey, A., Hodkinson, H. M., and Evans, G. J. The elderly in the wrong unit. *British Medical Journal,* 1968, *2*(16).

Mischel, W. Toward a cognitive social learning reconceptualization of personality. *Psychological Review,* 1973, *80*(4), 252–283.

Mischel, W. *Personality and assessment.* New York: John Wiley & Sons, Inc., 1968.

Mischara, B. L., and Kastenbaum, R. Wine in the treatment of long-term geriatric patients in mental hospitals. *Journal of the American Geriatrics Society,* 1974, *22,* 88–94.

Mischara, B. L., Robertson, B., and Kastenbaum, R. Self-injurious behavior in the elderly. *The Gerontologist,* 1973, *13,* 311–314.

Moos, R. H. Changing the social milieus of psychiatric treatment settings. *Journal of Applied Behavioral Science,* 1973, *9*(5), 575–593.

Morrice, J. K. W. *Crisis intervention: Studies in community care.* Oxford, England: Pergamon Press, 1976.

Motley, D. In *Older American Reports,* 1977, *1*(25), 7–8.

Mutschler, P. Factors affecting choice of and perseveration of social work with the aged. *The Gerontologist,* 1971, *11,* 231–241.

Neugarten, B. L., and Havighurst, R. J. (Eds.), *Social policy, social ethics, and the aging society.* Washington, D.C.: U.S. Government Printing Office, 1976.

Oberleder, M. Crisis therapy in mental breakdown of the aging. *The Gerontologist,* 1970, *10*(2), 111–114.

Orcutt, J. D. Societal reaction and the response to deviation in small groups. *Social Forces,* 1973, *52,* 259–267.

Ostrander, E. R. Research based nursing home design: An approach for planning environments for the aging. *International Journal of Aging and Human Development,* 1973, (4) 307–317.

Palmore, E. B., and Manton, K. Ageism compared to racism and sexism. *Journal of Gerontology,* 1973, *28,* 363–369.

Panyan, M., Boozer, H., and Morris, N. Feedback to attendants as a reinforcer for applying operant techniques. *Journal of Applied Behavior Analysis,* 1970, *3*(14).

Paul, G. L. Design tactics for outcome research in psychotherapy. In C. M. Franks (Ed.), *Behavior therapy: Appraisal and status.* New York: McGraw-Hill, 1969.

Peck, H. S., Kaplan, S. R., and Roman, M. Prevention, treatment and social action: A strategy of intervention in a disadvantaged urban area. *American Journal of Orthopsychiatry,* 1966, *36,* 57–69.

Perlich, D., and Atkins, A. *Effects of stated age on the differential diagnosis of Senile Dementia versus depression.* Unpublished manuscript. Montefiore Hospital, New York, New York, 1979.

Pfeiffer, E., and Busse, E. W. Mental disorders in later life—affective disorders; paranoid, neurotic, and situational reactions. In Busse & Pfeiffer (Eds.), *Mental Illness in Later Life.* Washington, D. C.-American Psychiatric Association, 1973.

Pfeiffer, E., and Davis, G. C. Determinants of sexual behavior in middle and old age. *Journal of the American Geriatrics Society,* 1972, *20*(4), 151–158.

Plutchik, R., McCarthy, M., Hall, B., and Silverberg, S. Evaluation of a comprehensive psychiatric and health care program for elderly welfare tenants in a single-room occupancy hotel. *Journal of the American Geriatrics Society,* 1973, *21*(10), 452–459.

Poser, E. G. The effect of therapist training on group therapeutic outcome. *Journal of Consulting Psychology,* 1966, *30,* 283–289.

Powell, R. R. Psychological effects of exercise therapy upon institutionalized geriatric mental patients. *Dissertation Abstract International,* 1972, *33*(6-A), 2771.

Quilitch, H. R. A comparison of three staff management procedures. *Journal of Applied Behavior Analysis,* 1975, *8,* 59–66.

Rappaport, J., Chinsky, J. M., and Cowen, E. L. *Innovations in helping chronic patients; College students in a mental institution.* New York: Academic Press, 1971.

Rathbone-McCuan, E., and Levenson, J. Impact of socialization therapy in a geriatric day-care setting. *The Gerontologist,* 1975, *15*(4), 338–342.

Reingold, J., and Wolk, R. L. Gerontological sheltered workshops for mentally impaired aged: Some tested hypotheses. *Industrial Gerontology,* 1974, *4,* 1–11.

Riessman, F. The paraprofessional and institutional change. In A. Gartner (Ed.), *Paraprofessionals and their performance.* New York: Praeger Publications, 1971.

Robinson, R. A. The prevention and rehabilitation of mental illness in the elderly. *Interdisciplinary Topics in Gerontology,* 1969, *3,* 89–102.

Rose, A. M., and Peterson, W. A. (Eds.), *Older people and their social world.* Philadelphia, Pennsylvania: F. A. Davis Co., 1965.

Rosenhan, D. L. The contextual nature of psychiatric diagnosis. *Journal of Abnormal Psychology,* 1975, *84*(5), 462–474.

Rosenhan, D. L. On being sane in insane places. *Science,* 1973, *179,* 250–258.

Rosow, I. Old age: One moral dilemma of an affluent society. *The Gerontologist,* 1962, *2,* 182–191.

Rubin, I. *Sexual life after sixty.* New York: Basic Books, 1965.

Ryan, W. *Blaming the victim.* New York: Vintage Books, 1971.

Sanoff, H., and Cohen, S. (Eds.), EDRA I: Proceedings of the first Environmental Design Research Association Conference, Raleigh, North Carolina, 1970.

Santore, A. F., and Diamond, H. The role of a community mental health center in developing services to the aging. *The Gerontologist,* 1974, *14,* 201–206.

Saunders, R., Smith, R. S., and Weinman, B. *Chronic psychosis and recovery: An experiment in socio-environmental therapy.* San Francisco, California: Jossey-Bass, 1967.

Scheff, T. (Ed.), *Mental illness and social processes.* New York: Harper & Row, 1967.

Schulz, R. The effects of control and predictability on the physical and psychological well-being of the institutionalized aging. *Journal of Personality and Social Psychology,* 1975, *33*(5), 563–573.

Schwartz, A. N. Planning micro-environments for the aged. In D. S. Woodruff and J. E. Birren (Eds.), *Aging: Scientific perspectives and social issues.* New York: Van Nostrand Co., 1975.

Settin, J. M. Comment: Some thoughts about diseases presenting as senility. *The Gerontologist,* 1978, *18*(1).

Settin, J. M. *Paraprofessional training and the aging.* Paper presented at Community Psychology: The Public Sector. Kings Park, New York: April 27, 1979.

Settin, J. M. *Program for training therapy aides to work with the aging.* Paper presented at Conference for Psychologists in New York State Service, Albany, New York: October 22, 1979.

Settin, J. M. *Client age, gender and class as determinants of clinicians' percep-*

tions: A study of labeling bias. Doctoral thesis, Department of Psychology, State University of New York at Stony Brook, 1979.

Settin, J. M. *Therapists' negative perceptions of aging clients.* Paper presented at Annual Meeting of Gerontological Society of America, San Diego, California, November, 1980.

Settin, J. M., and Julius, N. CRISIS Training: A counseling, referral, and information service for seniors. Unpublished manuscript, Department of Psychology, State University of New York at Stony Brook, 1977.

Selye, H. A. Stress and aging. *Journal of the American Geriatrics Society,* 1970, *18*(9), 669–690.

Shaie, K. W. Translations in gerontology from lab to life. *American Psychologist,* 1974, *29,* 802–807.

Shapiro, A. A pilot program in music therapy with residents of a home for the aged. *The Gerontologist,* 1969, *9*(2,1), 128–133.

Shattin, L., Kotter, W., and Longmore, G. Psycho-social prescription for music therapy in hospitals. *Diseases of the Nervous System,* 1967, *28*(4), 231–233.

Shore, H. Designing a training program for understanding sensory losses in aging. *The Gerontologist,* 1976, *16*(2), 157–165.

Siegel, J. S. Some demographic aspects of aging in the United States. In A. M. Ostfield and D. C. Gibson (Eds.), *Epidemiology of aging,* 1972, Bethesda, Maryland: DHEW Publication No. 75–711.

Silverstone, B., and Winter, L. The effects of introducing a heterosexual living space. *The Gerontologist,* 1975, *17,* 83–85.

Smith, J. B. Florida's gray power in action. *Newsday,* January 3, 1979, p. 41.

Snyder, L. H. An exploratory study of patterns of social interaction organization, and facility design in three nursing homes. *Aging and Human Development,* Spring 1973.

Sobey, F. *The nonprofessional revolution in mental health.* New York: Columbia University Press, 1970.

Solomon, K. *The development of stereotypes of the elderly: Toward a unified hypothesis.* Paper presented at 31st Annual Meeting of Geriatrics Society, 1978.

Sommer, R., and Ross, H. Social interaction on a geriatric ward. *International Journal of Social Psychology,* 1958, *3,* 128–133.

Stamford, B. A. Psychological effects of training upon institutionalized geriatric men. *Journal of Gerontology,* 1972, *27,* 451–455.

Steinfeld, E. *Acting toward the environment in old age.* Paper presented at 5th Annual SAGE Conference, Buffalo, New York, October 1977.

Stirner, F. W. The transportation needs of the elderly in a large urban environment. *The Gerontologist,* 1978, *18*(2), 207–211.

Stone, V., and Kranz, D. S. *Reactions to uncontrollable events in young and old persons.* Paper presented at Gerontological Society Meeting, New York, New York, 1976.

Stone, G., and Vance, A. Instructions, modeling, and rehearsal: Implications for training. *Journal of Counseling Psychology*, 1976, *23*, 272–279.

Taulbee, R. R., and Folsom, J. C. Reality orientation for geriatric patients. Hospital and Community Psychiatry, 1966, *17*, 23–25.

Thompson, L. W., and Marsh, G. R. Psychophysiological studies of aging. In C. Eisdorfer and E. P. Lawton (Eds.), *Psychology of Adult Development and Aging*, Washington, D.C.-American Psychological Association, 1973.

Toseland, R., and Rasch, J. Factors contributing to older persons' satisfaction with their communities. *The Gerontologist*, 1978, *18*(4), 395–402.

U.S. Vital Statistics of the United States, Vol. II, Mortality, Part A. Washington, D.C.: U.S. Public Health Service, 1968.

Vasquez, J., and Makinodan, T. Aging and the immune system. A brief summary of current knowledge. In A. M. Ostfeld and D. C. Gibson (Eds.), *Epidemiology of Aging*, U.S. Department of Health, Education and Welfare, DHEW Publication #(NIH) 75–711, 1972.

Wahl, C. W. Psychological treatment of the dying patient. In R. H. Davis (Ed.), *Dealing with Death*, Ethel Percy Andrus Gerontology Center, University of Southern California, 1973.

Wang, H. S. Special diagnostic procedures—the evaluation of brain impairment. In Busse and Pfeiffer (Eds.), *Mental illness in later life*. Washington, D.C.: American Psychiatric Association, 1973.

Wang, H. S., Obrist, W. D., and Busse, E. W. Neurophysiological correlates of the intellectual function. In E. Palmore (Ed.), *Normal aging II*, Durham, North Carolina: Duke University Press, 1974.

Wechsler, D. The measurement and appraisal of adult intelligence. Baltimore, Maryland: Williams & Wilkins, 1958.

Weg, R. B. The changing physiology of aging. In R. H. Davis (Ed.), *Aging prospects and issues*. Los Angeles, California: University of Southern California Press, 1973.

Weisman, A. D. *On dying and denying*, New York: Behavioral Publication, 1972.

Weissert, W. G. Two models of geriatric day care. *The Gerontologist*, 1976, *16*(5), 420–427.

Wershow, H. J. Reality orientation for gerontologists: Some thoughts about senility. *The Gerontologist*, 1977, *17*, 297–302.

Whanger, A. D., and Busse, E. W. Pessimism in treatment or lack of it. In B. Wolman (Ed.), *The therapist's handbook*, New York: Van Nostrand Reinhold Co., 1976.

Whanger, A. D., and Wang, H. S. Vitamin B_{12} deficiency in normal aged and elderly psychiatric patients. In E. Palmore (Ed.), *Normal aging II*, Durham, N.C.-Duke University Press, 1974.

Wolff, K. Comparison of group and individual psychotherapy with geriatric patients. *Diseases of the Nervous System*, 1967, *28*(6), 384–386.

Yalom, I. D., and Terrazas, F. Group therapy for psychotic elderly patients. *American Journal of Nursing,* 1968, *68*(8), 1960–1964.

Zerbe, M., and Hickey, T. Self-maintenance skills: A continuing education program for geriatric nursing. *Journal of Gerontological Nursing,* 1974, *1*(2), 5–9.

Zax, M., and Specter, G. A. *An introduction to community psychology,* New York: John Wiley & Sons, Inc., 1974.

PROGRAM FOR TRAINING THERAPY AIDES IN AGING

MODULAR EXPERIENTIAL TRAINING IN AGING

   I. Stereotypes
  II. Loneliness
 III. Nonverbal Communication
  IV. Verbal Communication—Listening
   V. Verbal Communication—Feedback
  VI. Sensory Deprivation
 VII. Touching
VIII. Loss of Mobility
  IX. Learned Helplessness
   X. Sexuality
  XI. Death
 XII. Interviewing—Reflecting
XIII. Interviewing—Probing
 XIV. Orientation to New Setting
  XV. Invasion of Privacy
 XVI. Territoriality

Most training programs focus on task-oriented behavior. This is particularly true in programs for geriatric clients, since the nursing contingent forms a strong influence on curricular material. The focus in this training program is instead upon client-oriented behavior. Using modeling, role playing, and immediate feedback, therapy aides working on a geriatric admissions unit of a large psychiatric center received on-the-job training in topics of particular relevance in gerontology. The modular training situations are designed for paraprofessionals who may not have didactic gerontology training prior to entering the job situation, and who are largely involved in supportive and often custodial tasks with the clients. Helping skills, such as warmth, empathy, interest, and belief in the client's ability to form meaningful relationships with the therapy aide, form the basis for the program. Modules are based upon special problems of the aging, such as physical disability, loneliness, and sensory deprivation, which have wide application in chronic as well as acute cases in nursing homes, medical hospitals, and other health-related facilities and may be readily adapted for use in community settings.

Module I: Stereotypes

Objective:	To provide insight and awareness into expectancies concerning the process of aging.
Exercise:	Trainees are induced with eyes closed into relaxed state through five-minute relaxation exercises. They are then told they will be projecting themselves at successive developmental stages, beginning with the age of 45 and by decade going to age 95.
Discussion:	a) What difficulties were experienced while trying to project their future aging?
	b) What physical changes were observed at each stage?
	c) Was the future seen as being alone or with other people, and what person did the trainee most identify with during aging?

> d) Where did trainees view themselves as living? What were they doing at the age of 80?
>
> e) How differently do younger versus older trainees perceive their futures?
>
> f) Do future perceptions reflect a view of old age that is more negative or more positive, and is this a realistic perception?

Module II: Loneliness

Objective:	To promote insight into causes of loneliness and to experience the outcome of sharing loneliness with others.
Exercise:	In a circle, trainees will recollect their single most lonely time, and relive the feelings alone, with closed eyes, for several moments. Then, trainees will write a brief account of the situation and share with group members.
Discussion:	a) What emotions were evoked while trainees relived their own experience and while others were describing their own experiences?
	b) What similarities were observed in the loneliness situations?
	c) How might loneliness be more common or less common, for the aging than younger individuals?
	d) How do loneliness and social isolation differ, and which most accurately characterizes the aging?

Module III: Nonverbal Communication

Objective:	To demonstrate the impact of nonverbal behavior from both a giving and a receiving perspective on communications with the aging client.
Exercise:	Trainees stand in group circle (no larger than 10 persons), and each person in turn stands in the

middle, goes to each group member and lets them know nonverbally that they like them.

Discussion:
a) What were the specific nonverbal behaviors noted by group members?

b) What was the impact of the behavior in question on the giver and receiver, e.g., which role was most comfortable?

c) How did participants experience being touched?

d) What body-protecting behaviors were noticed?

Module IV: Verbal Communication—Listening

Objective:
To promote sensitivity to the effect that selective listening has on accuracy of perceptions about an aging person's communications.

Exercise:
Trainees form dyads where they alternate roles in speaking and listening. Speaker A takes five minutes to relate his or her entire autobiography (reminiscing). Speaker B then relates back as much information, in detail, as is recalled while Speaker A assesses the retelling for accuracy. Roles are exchanged.

Discussion:
a) How well was the listener able to relate an accurate account?

b) How did monitoring the time affect attentive listening?

c) What behavior did the listener show speaker to indicate comprehension and continued interest?

d) Was the speaker comfortable disclosing personal information? What did listener do to facilitate disclosure?

e) How can silence on the speakers' parts be dealt with?

Module V: Verbal Communication—Feedback

Objective:	To facilitate giving and receiving effective feedback with the aging person.
Exercise:	Trainees sit in small groups (no larger than 10 persons), where they each take turns sitting in the center of the group while outside group members tell the center person, in turn, three things they each like about him or her. The center person may not respond verbally. The group continues until all members have functioned in the feedback-receiving role.
Discussion:	a) How did the feedback receiver feel about the feedback (e.g., was it uncomfortable to receive a compliment)?
	b) Did the feedback seem genuine?
	c) How clear was the feedback (e.g., did it focus on the specific rather than the general)?
	d) Were there contradictions in the feedback givers' verbal and nonverbal behavior?
	e) How comfortable did the feedback givers appear?

Module VI: Sensory Deprivation

Objective:	To provide experience of sensory deprivation (visual sense).
Materials:	Blindfold
Exercise:	Trainees form dyads; partner A is blindfolded; partner B will take A on walk for 20 minutes, during which time there should be no verbal interaction. Partner B must indicate positive aspects of environment to be experienced by partner A as well as dangers. Roles are reversed.

Discussion: a) What specific anxieties were experienced by
                      blindfolded partner A?
                   b) Were the nonvisual aspects of the environment
                      experienced differently?
                   c) What were some of the nonverbal cues used by
                      partner B to direct blindfolded partner A?
                   d) As time passed, did partner A's degree of com-
                      fort increase or decrease?

Module VII: Touching

Objective: To foster awareness of the aging person's need to
                   be touched.
Exercise: Trainees will sit back to back in dyads without
                   touching, and each in turn will relate to the other
                   one thing that is frightening about growing old.
                   Then, after turning to face each other, the same
                   fear will be repeated, this time touching.
Discussion: a) How did each person feel about being touched?
                   b) Were differences in the pressure of touch
                      noticed as the fearful concern was related?
                   c) How did facing one another affect the degree of
                      comfort?
                   d) To what degree did touching facilitate, or im-
                      pede, comfort?

Module VIII: Loss of Mobility

Objective: To increase ability to relate subjectively to the
                   feelings experienced by the immobilized aging
                   client.
Materials: Geriatric chairs with lock-arm restraints, or
                   wheelchairs.
Exercise: Each trainee is instructed to be immobilized in a
                   geriatric chair or wheelchair for fifteen minutes,
                   preferably in a work setting where other people

are similarly confined. Following immobilization, trainees should write a two-page account of
their experiences, paying attention to their
thought processes during restraint.

Discussion: a) What did trainees notice about the passage of
time?

b) How did trainees perceive others in similar
situations from their position of immobility?

c) What did trainees notice about nonconfined
persons (e.g., staff)?

d) Did the immobility have any effect on need
gratification?

e) What did trainees notice about their physical
comfort?

f) Was there any increase in daydreaming or fan-
tasizing as a result of immobility?

Module IX: Learned Helplessness

Objective: To promote understanding of the interaction between dependency behavior and infantalization.

Exercise: Sometime prior to group meeting, two trainees
are instructed to alternate in feeding each other an
entire meal. The receiver may not use hands or
arms. Meal should encompass different food tex-
tures.

Discussion: a) Was it more difficult to be on the giver or the
receiver end?

b) Describe how the rate of feeding affected the
enjoyment of the food.

c) While being fed, were instructions communicated to the giver and if so did giver heed the
instructions?

d) What feelings were evoked for the giver concerning the experience of feeding an adult a
whole meal?

e) Imagine that all meals had to be taken in this passive manner, and the effect this would have on feelings about both self and the caretaker.

Module X: Sexuality

Objective: To explore feelings about sexuality and aging.

Exercise: A trainee aide enters semi-private room and finds female occupants cuddled together in the same bed. The trainee tells occupants, "That kind of thing isn't allowed here," and in a punitive tone of voice orders Ms. A. back to her own bed.

Discussion: a) What assumption did the trainee make in this situation?

b) How did these assumptions relate to the trainee's attitudes toward sexuality?

c) Are sex and sexuality the same thing?

d) What would have been an alternate interpretation of clients' behavior?

e) What does this alternative interpretation indicate about the needs of the two clients?

Module XI: Death

Objective: To recognize feelings concerning death.

Exercise: Trainees are asked to write their own eulogy. It should be at least a page long, and should include how and where they died. Participants then share their eulogy with others.

Discussion: a) What were feelings while writing eulogy?

b) List feelings and discuss.

c) Given a choice of how to die a "happy" death, what scene would be imagined?

d) What would be felt if dying in an institution?

Module XII: Interviewing—Reflecting

Objective:	To demonstrate nonevaluative communication during information exchange with the aging.
Exercise:	Mr. D., a 78-year-old man, has been institutionalized for five years. He is a "cooperative patient" and even assists the staff with their work with other clients. He appears carefree, bright, amiable, but refuses to discuss personal matters about his past life. When questioned, he becomes mildly agitated, noncommittal, and seeks to change the subject by joking. One trainee paraprofessional plays role of client, one of interviewer.
Discussion:	a) Differentiate between statements that can be answered directly by interviewer and statements that require reflecting or mirroring.
	b) What feelings are aroused in the interviewer as he or she reflects?
	c) What feelings are aroused in the interviewee as he or she hears the interviewer reflecting?
	d) At what point in the interview can reflection be carried one step further to interpretation, and what dangers lie in interpretation?

Module XIII: Interviewing—Probing

Objective:	To assist paraprofessionals in maximizing information exchange during interview with the aging.
Exercise:	Trainee will observe a five-minute interview with an aging client (it can be videotaped or role-played) in order to identify leading responses, including influential questions, and advice giving.
Discussion:	a) What sort of interviewing style fits best with

information-seeking-type interview? Direct? Reflective? Does it depend on the client or his or her particular situation?

b) What, if any, personal questions should be asked regarding past drug involvement, alcoholism, injuries, prior hospitalizations, etc.

c) How does one get started on an interview? What role do you see yourself as having? Protective? Demanding?

d) What can silence mean during an interview? Is it always negative or something to be avoided? How can it be used to spark further information gathering?

e) How aware are you of the client's feelings during the interview? How can one handle hostility to the interview/interviewer?

f) What are your feelings as an interviewer?

g) What sort of "blocks" can occur in the interviewing process?

Module XIV: Orientation to New Setting

Objective: To foster awareness concerning the impact of an unfamiliar environment on the aging clients (e.g., external versus internal causes of behavior).

Exercise: Mrs. J., an ambulatory 68-year-old woman, was admitted to N.H. at 10:00 a.m., brought in by her family who left shortly after her admission. She was given her room, shown where her bed was. She did not see anyone until after 12:30 p.m., at which time she was sitting in her chair crying and incontinent of urine. Client indicated that she had not been incontinent at home but was often confused. What would be the best approach for the trainee coming into client's room? One paraprofessional trainee plays role of client, other plays role of staff.

Discussion: a) Was client shown location of bathroom?

b) Was client introduced to staff members and advised how to obtain assistance?

c) Was client given a schedule of activities, including mealtimes?

Module XV: Invasion of Privacy

Objective: To communicate feelings evoked by sudden invasion of privacy.

Exercise: Trainees will empty out their pockets, pocketbooks, briefcases, or wallets onto a table in view of others.

Discussion: a) What specific response was elicited by this invasion of privacy (e.g. anger, pleasure, etc.)?

b) Of the persons trainees know personally, with whom would they feel most comfortable doing this exercise?

c) Why would it be particularly important to request an aging person's need for privacy.

Module XVI: Territoriality

Objective: To acquaint trainees with the fact that each individual has his or her own personal space.

Exercise: Trainees pair up and, beginning from the outer boundaries of the room, approach each other gradually until they reach a degree of discomfort.

Discussion: a) What differences can be noted in the distance between pairs?

b) When was discomfort felt by trainees?

c) How did the trainee react to this discomfort?

d) How did trainees know when they were invading someone's personal space? What behavioral cues were noted?

e) How can this information be utilized when dealing with elderly clients?

CRISIS TRAINING

The CRISIS Training program (Settin and Julius, 1977) was designed to span ten weeks, conforming to one semester, and to provide at least 20 intensified hours of Hotline training in phone counseling, referral, information giving, with an aging population. Volunteers were recruited through the State University of New York at Stony Brook paper; word-of-mouth volunteers and came primarily from social welfare, psychology, and sociology departments. Committed volunteers formed a core of approximately 15 persons, predominantly female, although as many as 30 persons attended any given training session. No volunteer who missed more than two sessions was allowed to continue on to the implementation stage the following semester. Each session combined didactic with experiential training techniques, relying heavily on role playing and multi-media educational materials (films and cassettes on aging). Group discussion was encouraged, with group leader acting as facilitator rather than instructor. Each trainee received worksheets during sessions, to be entered into a training packet designed to later provide trainee with refresher-guidelines. Selected worksheets are presented, following the training outline.

CRISIS TRAINING OUTLINE

I. Personal Motivation and Goals
   a. Experiencing aging
   b. Forming helping relationships (worksheet #1)
II. Prevention
   a. Identifying helping sources in the community (worksheet #2)
   b. Evaluating resources
III. Communication
   a. Assertive Phone Technique (worksheet #3)
   b. Identifying the target population (worksheet #4)
IV. Interviewing (Part 1)
   a. Listening and attending
   b. Probing neutrally (worksheet #5)
V. Interviewing (Part 2)
   a. Giving effective feedback (worksheet #6)
   b. Using self-involvement
VI. Referral
   a. Role of the paraprofessional
   b. Ethical and legal responsibilities
   c. Discriminating crisis situations
VII. Facts About Aging
   a. Dispelling myths
   b. Relating stereotypes to personal experience
VIII. Special Problems of Aging
   a. Identifying environmental, community-specific problems (worksheet #7)
   b. Depression: Major Problem of the Aging (worksheet #8)
IX. Dealing with Problematic Calls
   a. Hostility
   b. Annoyance
   c. Suicide
X. Summary—Five Stages of Phone Interviewing

WORKSHEET #1

Forming Helping Relationships:
Characteristics of Effective Interactions

1) Demonstrating *respect* to the client: Respect for the client and the client's world involves a sincere interest. This is communicated by the manner in which the client is attended by the paraprofessional and by putting aside outside interference as much as possible while the interaction is occurring. Address the client by the surname, e.g., good morning, Mr. Smith. In this way, the client will feel that what is important to the client is important to the paraprofessional.

2) *Accepting* the client: Acceptance actually means treating the client as an equal. This is why we refer to people as clients rather than patients. Never disregard the client's thoughts and feelings because they differ from one's own. This involves maintaining an openness and willingness to understand the client. Acceptance also involves maintaining an unbiased attitude toward the client no matter what preconceived stereotyped notions have been formed.

3) *Listening* to the client: Listening involves not only hearing the surface meaning of what the client is saying, but also attending to the tone of voice, expressions, and gestures employed by the client. This is called "listening with the third ear," and is like detective work in the sense that the paraprofessional has to pick up disguised underlying meanings.

4) Genuine *liking* for the client: The paraprofessional who truly enjoys other persons, and who has the ability to converse with many different types of persons, will be successful with clients. For example, if the paraprofessional is reserved or remote, how can the client be friendly? Similarly, if the paraprofessional is cautious, how can the client be unguarded?

5) *Empathy:* Empathy is perhaps the most important of all these characteristics. It describes a process whereby the paraprofessional attempts "to get in touch with" how the client is thinking, feeling, and acting by remaining open to receiving information (verbal or nonverbal). Although it is usually easier to establish an empathic "rapport" with the client who has a background of experience similar to yours, empathy can be achieved by

allowing other persons to talk freely about their experiences, their fears, their desires. A sensitivity to others is necessary for empathetic rapport. Empathy does not stop with understanding, but goes beyond to communicating this understanding to the client. Some response or gesture should be made that allows the client to feel that the paraprofessional has clearly understood the communication.

WORKSHEET #2

Identifying Helping Sources in the Community

To Hotline Members: The Recording Form indicates the basic content of information we need. It is not necessary for you to follow the format . . . just make sure you fill in all the information. answer any questions the contact may have in a professional manner. If contact wants more credentials, stress that you are basically seeking interested referral sources in order to make services available to aging persons who otherwise might not know their agency or service exists. If the contact is unwilling to cooperate and will not give you any information, fill out the Rater Judgment section of the form.

At the end of the conversation, get as much closure as to the real accessability of this service to us as you can., If the contact is cooperative, ask for descriptive materials to be forwarded c/o Joan Settin, Department of Psychology, SUNY at S.B., Stony Brook, N.Y. 11794.

Whether or not the contact has been pleasant, it is important that you end the phone interview on a nice note. Thank them for their time and assure those contacts that give a positive response that we will be in touch with them in September to provide them with more information about our service.

Do not provide the contact with a phone number, saying that we are now in the organizational stage and that it would be very difficult to get in touch at any of the currently available numbers.

The best approach is to be businesslike and assertive without sounding pushy. This means that you should be friendly but not under any circumstances sound like a student. What does a student sound like? People erroneously seem to expect students to be nonmembers of society in a way. They expect that they can put you off and that you won't persist, that you don't know what the world-outside-of-the-ivory-tower is really like, and that you are possibly doing a "school project." I'm sure you can all get around this by stressing how necessary such services are for a neglected group like the aging, and by using the academic "we" instead of "I." If you sound like you know what you're talking about, and particulary if you say things like, "when I worked with the aging in (some place) it emerged that one of the greatest problems was (housing)," the contact will be reassured that you are experienced and serious.

Recording Form

Name of agency_____

Name of contact (include title)_____

Address_____

Phone_____

Stated purpose of agency:

Community and population served _____

Years in operation _____

Percent of persons aged 65 and over utilizing service_____

Operating status (e.g., private, state)_____

Services currently offered relating to the aging:

How do these services differ from those of other agencies (e.g., what is special)?

Services in the planning stage:

Contact suggestions for follow-up (e.g., call Mr. _____ for further info):

Comments:

Send literature: Y   N   Willing to refer clients: Y   N

Favorable impression: Y   N   If No, why?

Recontact: Y   N   If Yes, specify time.

Recorded by_____Date_____

WORKSHEET #3

Assertive Phone Technique

"Hello,_____.

My name is_____and I sent you a letter last week about a project we are conducting for the community elderly. This project, called _____

_____, was briefly described in the letter. Have you any people to suggest to us whom we might be able to help?"

> If the contact has not read the letter, a copy of the letter will be posted for you to refer to in explanation.
>
> If you reach the contact's secretary or co-worker, ask when the contact is expected in and be sure to follow it up with:

"Perhaps you could help me."

> If the person you reach is not the contact, and says something like:

"I really don't think that Dr._____could be of any help to you,"

> say:

"Well, I'd very much like to speak with him/her about this, and it is rather important."

> If the contact is an agency or organization, start the conversation with the same format (Hello . . . etc.) but say:

"I'm wondering if you could connect me with someone who could give me some information about a liaison between your organization and the university on a project concerning the aging persons in the community."

> When you're connected, go through it all again and read the letter if you have to.
>
> There is no right or wrong way to do this. The main thing to remember is that you want to get to someone who can give you the information you're looking for. If you sound like you *expect* to be connected, you stand a better chance of getting through.

WORKSHEET #4

Identifying Target Population

"Hello, Mr./Ms._____. My name is _____
_____and I am calling from the Counseling, Referral and Informa-

tion Service for Seniors located in the Stony Brook area. Your name was suggested to us by _____. Our group has been formed in order to find out how we can help persons aged 65 and over in their communities by providing information and referral services. We are contacting persons like yourself to obtain some information about the problems confronting the aging in this community (such as transportation, food prices). All our information is private. If you know people who might need some assistance, would you be willing to give us their names so we could talk with them by phone? Thank you for speaking with us. If you have any questions, I'll be glad to try to answer them. Please feel free to call us at_____to obtain information or to talk with one of our counselors. Have a good day/evening."

Guidelines

1. Speak slowly, clearly, and loud enough, emphasizing key words.
2. Use a pleasant and considerate tone of voice, mentioning the person's name whenever possible to personalize the interaction.
3. Always be patient, and if asked to repeat phrases, do so as if it were the first time around.
4. Sound interested and earnest.
5. Stick to the point and be persistent, but never sound demanding, impatient, or pushy.
6. Gear your approach to the person you are speaking with (e.g., if the tone is formal, you might want to also be formal; but, if the tone is friendly and informal, don't get carried away).
7. Be brief and keep extra comments to a minimum.
8. Refrain from answering personal questions; if possible do not mention that you are a student but rather that you are from the Stony Brook area.
9. Try to get people to give pertinent information on the spot; otherwise, arrange a specific call-back time.
10. If you run into a real problem (e.g. threats, verbal abuse, inappropriate behavior), terminate the contact at once in a pleasant manner. Do not try to deal with this.
11. Do not try to answer technical questions about health, or to even speculate about the nature of a problem; this is what we are a referral service for.
12. After all of this, remember to be yourself and to trust that you have had sufficient experience to be able to "come across" successfully.

WORKSHEET #5

Probing

One of the most challenging aspects of phone work is helping the caller toward fuller communication. This may be accomplished by focusing on the feeling rather than the content of the interview. The most difficult part is getting the caller to put thoughts into words. At the beginning of the interview the caller's responses may be incomplete or unclear. This may be due to the fact that they may perceive certain topics to be embarrassing or socially unacceptable. Once rapport is established, however, the caller will give freer responses. Assuring the caller of the confidentiality of the communication will facilitate sharing of personal problems with the interviewer. It is important to recall that even the most thorough questionnaire format may produce first responses that are irrelevant. Yet, there is no such thing as a response that fails to tell you something. For example, note how the caller fails to answer the question but still gives important information:

I: Do you think you might become ill if you remain at home alone, or do you think you will be able to manage without becoming ill?

C: (1) I don't know what I'm going to do. (indecision, depression)

       (2) I wish I could get help with my health insurance. (financial problem)

Neutral Probing Techniques

Neutral probing may be used to stimulate a clearer response, or to prompt continuing responses from the caller. The caller often strays away from the central issue unless the interviewer keeps the caller "on target" by letting the caller know the interviewer is there. Making noises that indicate understanding, such as "Yes," "I see," or just plain "Um" will reinforce the caller in going ahead with the conversation. Repeating the caller's statement or repeating a question that has not been directly answered is a neutral technique that brings the caller back to the original thought without making judgment, inference, or interpretation. This technique is called reflecting or mirroring, and is an important technique to practice. In the following example, the caller responds to interviewer's question with a "feeling" statement, which the interviewer then mirrors in order to continue the thought:

I: Do you have anyone you can rely on in an emergency?

C: My sister, but she's never helped me before and there's no reason she'd be starting to help me now.

I: You say your sister has never helped you before?

Or, the interview may need further clarification, which is not forthcoming through mirroring. This can be done by giving the caller a subtle probe such as "I'm not sure I understood all of that. Could you explain it again to me please?" or "Could you tell me why you say that?"

Further examples of probes and methods of clarifying caller response:

I: Do you believe the war on poverty helped the population over the age of 65 in America?

C: That depends. (caller makes unclear, partial answer)

Possible probes to use:

I1. I'm not sure what you mean. Could you explain it to me?

I2. You said "that depends" . . . (pause) (Repeat question.)

I3. Could you give me a specific example?

C: Well, I"m just not certain that anything will be done to make this a better world.

I: You say you're not certain anything will help make things better, but just let me ask you this question. (Repeat original question.)

WORKSHEET #6

Effective Feedback

The most important thing to remember about effective feedback is that it should be helpful to the person receiving it. To be helpful, feedback must be given in such a way that the caller:

a) understands what is being said,

b) is able to accept the information (not necessarily agree with it). Feedback is information offered to persons you care about so they can see how well their behavior matches their intentions.

Some specific guidelines are:

1) First check out whether the person you want to speak to would like to have some feedback. Remember you have something to offer. If you think you must tell someone what you're thinking, despite his or her discomfort or unreadiness to listen, then there must be some other reason besides a sincere desire to help.

2) Timing: It helps if you speak up immediately. The more time that elapses between the behavior and your comments the harder it will be for the receiver of the feedback to know what you're talking about.

3) Descriptive—not evaluative—language: When you describe your own reaction and describe what you saw and heard, the client is free to use the information or not as he or she sees fit. Evaluative language usually makes people defensive and less able to hear. For example, "When you raised your voice and spoke louder, I felt nervous. I was afraid you thought I was stupid" NOT "You tried to push me around."

4) Be specific rather than general: Usually, if you tell someone he or she is "dominating" or being rude, it's not much help. A better way is to stick to concrete details, without inferences; to describe behavior, not personality or character. For example, "Just now when we were deciding on a plan, you interrupted three times." It also helps to be brief. Too many details can be overwhelming, and what happened last week or in another setting is not as important as when you observe right now.

5) Speak plain English: Technical language or psychological jargon is just confusing.

6) Try to speak in a warm, nonthreatening manner, i.e., consider the needs of the person on the receiving end.

7) Be sure to discuss what you've said until it's clear that both you and the receiver understand what you're saying.

WORKSHEET #7

Identifying Environmental Problems of the Aging

I. Activity Resources
   a. How easy is it to reach the food store, post office, police station, laundry, doctors' offices, bank?
   b. How many times per month are activity services used?
   c. Any trouble getting service from utility company, land-lord, police, repairpersons, garbage pick-up?

      d. Who does errands?

      e. If someone needs a place to stay for one night, is there location?

  II. Transportation

      a. Any trouble getting places?

      b. Own car, with current driver's license?

      c. Convenience: availability of bus, train?

      d. Are there friends, family to offer rides when needed?

      e. How many times per week out for walk?

  III. Home Environment

      a. How many years lived at present location?

      b. Is home in convenient, familiar neighborhood?

      c. Enough heat, hot water in home?

      d. Kitchen facilities accessible?

      e. Bathroom reachable from bedroom?

      f. Phone available?

      g. Presence of radio, TV?

      h. State of repair, safety features?

  IV. Recreation

      a. Nearest park, movie, library, church/temple, restaurant, community center.

      b. How often are above utilized?

      c. Special hobbies, sports?

      d. Belong to senior-citizen group?

      e. How often is recreation done away from home?

      f. Would consider education, courses, as recreation?

      g. Participation in volunteer activities?

  V. Social Interaction

      a. Live by self?

      b Prefer to live by self if possible?

      c How often are visits either in person or by phone with other persons?

      d. Do visitors ever come to house?

      e. How many times per week is next-door neighbor seen?

      f. How often is letter received from friend or family?

      g. Is there at least one person in whom to confide?

      h. Are there any pets?

      i. Are there groups regularly met with for planned activities?

      j. Are friends own age or mostly younger?

  VI. Family

      a. Marital status?

      b. Any children, grandchildren?

    c. Would live with relatives if could?
    d. How many times per year do close relatives get in touch?
    e. Does family care?
    f. Treated with respect by family? Is advice sought?
    g. Who is emotionally closest relative?
    h. Ever invited to visit family?

VII. Nutrition
    a. Are three meals per day eaten?
    b. Are meals satisfying and enough?
    c. Feel thirsty much during day?
    d. Do own cooking?
    e. Ever drink too much by self?
    f. How many cups coffee/tea drunk during day?
    g. Usually eat by self?
    h. Currently on diet for any reason?
    i. Take vitamins or dietary supplement regularly?

VIII. Economic
    a. Currently on fixed income, or can find employment if needed for income supplement?
    b. How many years ago stopped working?
    c. Interested in working now if could?
    d. Highest level of education?
    e. What was average yearly income when under 65?
    f. What is income now?
    g. Is Medicare/Medicaid adequate for medical expenses?
    h. Have savings, checking account?
    i. Contributing to someone else's income?
    j. Having trouble making ends meet?

IX. Adjustment
    a. Are most things boring and monotonous?
    b. Are interesting and pleasant things anticipated for the future?
    c. Looking back over life, is it felt that important things were attained?
    d. How satisfied with current life situation?
    e. Have plans been made to do things in next month?
    f. Are things as interesting as ever?
    g. Would change past if could?
    h. Belief in life after death?
    i. Best things about being current age?
    j. Improvements would like made in present life?

Depression: Major Problem of the Aging

What does it feel like to be depressed?

Cognitive—thoughts confused, difficulty concentrating.
Somatic—bodily reactions slowed, tension
Affective—some possible reactions:
  Feel miserable, irritable
  Calmness, sudden mood swings
  Cramped reactivity
  Regression and withdrawal (quiet or detached)
  Lack of spontaneity
  Outside seen as far away (each obstacle magnified)
  If severe, memory impaired (because of concentrating on
    problem)

Crisis approach

Focus on feelings
  Don't try to talk them out of depression
  Deal with isolation
  • Invite them to talk about themselves and respond with
    empathy
  • Explore who can turn to (may forget neighbor)
  • If depression is severe or recurring, *refer.*
Check out physical well-being
  When did they last eat, sleep?
  Is anything in need of doctor's attention
  Evaluate suicide potential, and *refer*
  • Hopelessness likely leads to person taking his life.
  • Anger leads to suicide as weapon.
  • Depression, followed by euphoria, may mean firming of
    decision to commit suicide.
Explore alternatives
  Friends, relatives who can help
  Therapy, counseling (only if client requests)
  Change (life situation or goals)

Relate back to external events

Explore recent history (if appropiate)

Mobilize anger and constructive assertion

If anger underlies depression, let person know it's okay to verbalize feelings of resentment, anger. May be due to unalterable situations:

Death or loss of loved one.

- Grief at loss
- Other feelings not resolved (i.e. anger, guilt)

Terminal illness/or physical disability.

Normal aging and other hormonal or biochemical changes, such as sensory loss associated with age.

Kids leave home.

Relocation.

Retirement.

Living on fixed income.

INDEX